The Expectant Mother's Guide to

Prescription a on

Drugs, Vitam ies,

and Herbal Products

D0462225

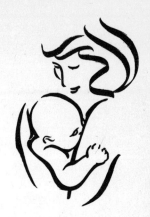

THE EXPECTANT MOTHER'S GUIDE TO

Prescription and Nonprescription

Drugs, Vitamins, Home Remedies,

and Herbal Products

DONALD L. SULLIVAN, R.Ph., Ph.D.

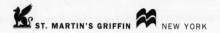

ST. MARTIN'S GRIFFIN   NEW YORK

www.stmartins.com

Book design by Gretchen Achilles

Library of Congress Cataloging-in-Publication Data

Sullivan, Donald L.
    The expectant mother's guide to prescription and nonprescription drugs, vitamins, home remedies, and herbal products / Donald L. Sullivan.—1st ed.
        p. cm.
      ISBN 0-312-25190-4
      1. Obstetrical pharmacology—Popular works. 2. Pregnant women—Health and hygiene. I. Title.

    RG528 .S85 2001
    618.2'4—dc21   2001041955

FIRST EDITION: November 2001

10 9 8 7 6 5 4 3 2 1

To my loving wife, Amy; my parents, Jan and Donna Sullivan; and my brother, Jerry Sullivan, for all the love and support you gave me in writing this book. I will never forget all you have done for me. I could not have accomplished this book without you.

Note to Readers

This book was written to provide selected information to the public concerning frequently prescribed medications. Research about prescription drugs is an ongoing process; side effects and adverse reactions to particular drugs sometimes continue to be reported to the FDA after a drug has been approved for use in the general market. As a result, what we know about the drugs discussed in this book could change with time and future research. The reader should also keep in mind that we have included information on open questions, debates, and controversies regarding drug use and safety that have been reported in medical journals and major periodicals. Our aim here is simply to report that these concerns exist, not to take a position on the scientific validity of any one claim.

Readers should bear in mind that this book is not intended to be used for self-diagnosis or self-treatment; they should consult their doctor about any and all medical problems. Readers should never stop taking a prescription drug or alter the dosage or dosing schedule without first consulting their physicians. Neither the publisher nor the author takes responsibility for possible consequences from any treatment action or application of medicine or preparation by a person reading or following the information in this book.

The fact that an organization is listed in the book as a potential source of information does not mean that the author or publisher endorses any of the information it may provide or recommendations it may make.

Contents

Acknowledgments

I would like to thank my family for all their love and support while I was writing this book. I would like to thank one person in particular—my wife, Amy—for all her help. She spent dozens of hours editing the text, working on the computer, and doing many other little things that were greatly appreciated. I would like to thank Crystal Hall and Sara Jutte for all their help and research in preparing this book as well. I would also like to thank my agent, Rick Balkin, for his special contribution. His guidance and knowledge in the world of publishing are worth more than words can describe. Finally, I would like to thank Heather Jackson Silverman and St. Martin's Press for recognizing this book's potential.

Introduction

Jacqueline Adams, a computer programmer for Comtex Inc., has one month to go until she delivers her first child. While working on a sophisticated computer program one day, she develops a nasty tension headache. She cannot remember the last time she had one. She sits in her cubicle and thinks about what she can take to get rid of it. She knows that aspirin reduces the risk of heart attacks and strokes, as well as relieving pain, so Jacqueline assumes it's okay to take some. She asks a coworker for some, and is given two 500mg aspirin tablets. Half an hour later her headache is gone. What she doesn't know, however, is that aspirin should never be taken during the last trimester of pregnancy, because it has been found to cause stillbirth or life-threatening heart abnormalities in some infants. Jacqueline should have taken acetaminophen (Tylenol®) instead. Taking aspirin is a very common mistake made by pregnant women.

Tina Stambaugh is a health fanatic. She's three months pregnant and in perfect health. She exercises on her bike four times a week, eats a well-balanced diet, doesn't drink or smoke, avoids caffeine, and gets plenty of rest. She's doing everything she can to ensure that her child will be born healthy. Tina also takes large amounts of vitamins to make sure that her baby is receiving all the nutrients it needs. In fact, Tina has been taking large quantities of vitamins for the past five years. She's not aware that some of these can adversely affect her unborn child. Large doses of vitamin A can cause heart abnormalities or spontaneous abortion; large doses of vitamin D can cause mental retardation or cardiovascular disease; and large doses of iron can cause various gastrointestinal problems in the fetus as well as congenital anomalies.

Joan Dysert, five months pregnant, develops a painful sinus infection. It's the weekend, and she assumes she won't be able to get in touch with her doctor. She has some year-old tetracycline (an antibiotic) left over from her last sinus infection, and remembers that it really did the trick. Joan also has friends who took antibiotics for sore throats and sinus infections when they were pregnant. She erroneously concludes that it must be safe to take the tetracycline. What she doesn't realize is that this drug can cause deformed teeth, tooth discoloration, underdeveloped tooth enamel of the teeth in unborn children, and a whole host of other serious problems in the fetus.

Julie Robbins has been breast-feeding her baby for four months. Recently, she has begun to suffer from anxiety attacks. She made an appointment with her family doctor. The doctor prescribed Valium 5mg three times a day for three weeks. Soon after beginning the Valium, Julie noticed that her baby was very lethargic, listless, and drowsy all the time. She became concerned and called her pediatrician. What Julie did not know was that Valium passes into the breast milk in significant concentrations and can cause those types of adverse effects in breast-feeding infants.

These are all very real examples of women who want the best for their children and would do anything to protect them. Yet, one small mistake could result in dire consequences and serious birth defects. Health care professionals often fail to adequately explain the risks of taking prescription or over-the-counter drugs, large quantities of vitamins, and other chemicals to their pregnant patients. They don't tell women that there are risks as well as benefits associated with taking even something as common as aspirin when you're pregnant. The unborn child shares the mother's blood supply, nutrients, oxygen, and so on. Everything an expectant mother ingests eventually makes its way to the fetus. Every mother wants her baby to be born healthy. This book will help each mother give her unborn baby a greater-than-average chance of that.

The book begins with a chapter that discusses the entire pregnancy process from conception to birth. This will help the reader understand the physical changes a woman's body is undergoing. Chapter 1 then discusses how medications, vitamins, herbal products, and the like affect the fetus. A discussion is provided regarding the Food and Drug Administration's (FDA) classification system of risk from medications, vitamins, herbal products, toxins, etc. Chapter 1 concludes with a general discussion of the dangers of medications and chemicals that pass into the breast milk and their potential adverse affects on the infant.

Chapters 2 through 6 provide in-depth discussions of individual prescription drugs, over-the-counter drugs, herbal products, vitamins, chemicals, and toxins and their potential effects on the fetus during pregnancy and in the infant while breast-feeding. Products in each chapter are arranged alphabetically by brand name. Each entry will include the federal government's rating of risk. This is a rating the Food and Drug Administration has assigned to the product based on its potential adverse effect on the fetus. Next, a visual risk scale is provided to further illustrate the potential risk to the fetus. This scale was derived from the FDA rating and research reports that have documented potential risk to the fetus of a particular product. The visual risk scale may indicate more risk in some instances than the FDA rating. The author considered other published studies and case reports when assigning a risk rating to a particular drug. Next, a short discussion of the potential adverse effects on the fetus is presented. Finally, each entry closes with a short discussion on the potential of the product to pass into the breast milk. For readers who want more information on the risk to the fetus of a specific product or chemical, the Appendix provides a list of additional reference sources.

The Expectant Mother's Guide to Prescription and Nonprescription Drugs, Vitamins, Home Remedies, and Herbal Products

CHAPTER 1

Pregnancy and Breast-feeding: What Every Mother Needs To Know

Diagnosis

The first sign of pregnancy is usually a missed menstrual period. However, some women may have other symptoms of pregnancy before they miss their first period. These may include morning sickness, tender breasts, enlarged breasts, more frequent urination, and darkening of the nipples. Pregnancy is most often confirmed by detecting the presence of human chorionic gonadotropin (HCG) in the blood or urine. Some laboratories are sophisticated enough to detect levels of HCG in the blood 7 to 9 days after the egg is fertilized by the sperm. However, most blood tests confirm pregnancy 6 to 10 days after the egg has implanted itself into the uterus, which is usually within the first week after a missed period. These tests use radioimmunoassay (RIA) or enzyme-linked immunosorbent assay (ELISA) techniques to confirm pregnancy. They are more accurate and reliable than a urine pregnancy test.

Home pregnancy tests use monoclonal antibodies to detect the presence of HCG in the urine. These tests can detect the presence of HCG in the urine one to two weeks after the first day of a missed period. Home pregnancy tests have become much more reliable in recent years. When used correctly, they are 97 percent accurate. A false negative result, in which the patient is pregnant but the test indicates she is not, can occur up to 25 percent of the time. Usually these false negative results are due to errors in following the directions of the test. If a woman receives a negative result from a home pregnancy test and still believes she is pregnant, she should retest in about a week, or see her doctor. False positive results, in which the patient is not pregnant but the test indicates she is, occur less than 4 percent of the time. Women taking birth control pills (oral contraceptives) will not receive false positive results. If a woman receives a positive result from a home pregnancy test, she should assume she is pregnant and make an appointment to see her doctor.

The one problem with home pregnancy tests is their inability to consistently detect an ectopic pregnancy, implantation of the egg in an area outside the uterus like the fallopian tubes. Home pregnancy tests fail to detect 50 percent of all ectopic pregnancies. Women who experience negative results and the continued absence of menses should make an appointment with their doctor to rule out an ectopic pregnancy.

Tips for Using Home Pregnancy Kits

1. Kits with sticks on which the woman urinates are easier to use than those by which the urine must be collected in a cup.

2. Follow the directions carefully.

3. Wait until at least the second or third day after menses was supposed to begin before you test.

4. Use a morning urine sample for the test. The levels of HCG, if present, will be concentrated at this time.

5. Test the urine sample immediately after collection. If you cannot test the sample at this time, place the sample

in the refrigerator. Once the sample has been placed in the refrigerator, you must allow the sample to warm to room temperature before testing.

6. Any sediment or solids in the sample should not be mixed or shaken up. Let them settle on the bottom of the collection cup.

Calculating a Due Date

Now that you know you are pregnant, the next question is usually, when am I due? The normal length of pregnancy is 267 days from the time a woman's egg is fertilized by the sperm, or 280 days from the first day of the last menstrual period (about 40 weeks). There are various charts and tables that allow doctors to estimate the due date of the baby but it is usually confirmed by ultrasound. Women can use a mathematical formula to estimate their own due date called Nagele's rule. To calculate the due date using Nagele's rule, take the date of the first day of the last menstrual period, subtract three months, and add 7 days. For example: If the first day of the last menstrual period was July 10, you subtract 3 months from July 10 and add 7 days (July 10 - 3 months = April 10 + 7 days = April 17 as the expected due date). This method is usually accurate to within 2 weeks of delivery and works best in women with a normal 28-day cycle.

Development of the Baby

Many expectant parents do not realize that a baby actually begins growing and developing even before the egg implants itself into the uterus, but let's start the story with the point at which fertilization occurs. Fertilization of the mother's egg by the sperm occurs in the fallopian tubes. Within 24 hours of fertilization, the egg, now called an embryo, begins to grow and multiply. This initial growth and development occurs for about 6 days as the embryo continues its journey down the fallopian tubes to the uterus. During these first 6 days, the embryo receives its nutrition from secretions released from the mother's cells that line the fallopian tubes.

At about day 6, the embryo arrives at the uterus and floats freely, receiving its nutrients from the secretions produced by the lining of the uterus. On or about day 7, the embryo attaches itself to the lining of the uterus and then begins implanting itself into the endometrium. The embryo secretes enzymes that erode a small portion of the uterine lining. By day 10, the embryo has implanted itself firmly and completely into the endometrium.

After implantation, the amnion begins to develop and will eventually surround the entire embryo. This is also referred to as the amniotic sac. The space between this sac and the embryo is filled with clear fluid called amniotic fluid. This keeps the embryo moist and provides a cushion against mechanical injury. The placenta is also beginning to develop about the same time as the amnion. The placenta is the organ of exchange or pathway between the mother and baby. It is the organ by which nutrients are passed to the baby from the mother, as well as the channel by which waste is removed from the baby to be excreted by the mother. The placenta also secretes hormones such as estrogen, progesterone, and HCG.

Estrogen stimulates the uterus to enlarge, the breasts to grow and develop to prepare for breast-feeding, and increases the elasticity of the pelvis in preparation for birth. Progesterone provides early nutrition for the embryo and prevents the uterus from contracting, which prevents spontaneous abortions, and may also help prepare the breasts for breast-feeding. Probably the most important hormone secreted by the placenta is HCG. HCG signals the body that pregnancy has begun and causes additional release of estrogen and progesterone by the body. This action further stimulates the endometrium and placenta to continue developing. If HCG was not present, the endometrium would begin to deteriorate, disintegrate, and be sloughed off along with the embryo, and menses would begin. Therefore, HCG is essential for a pregnancy to be maintained by the body.

The stages of pregnancy are divided into three equal periods or trimesters, each containing three months. The first trimester is months 1 through 3, the second, months 4 through 6, and the third, months 7 through 9. From the time the egg is fertilized through the end of the eighth week of pregnancy, the developing organism is referred to as an embryo; from the ninth week to delivery the baby is referred to as a fetus. At nine weeks, the embryo actually contains most of its important body parts and that's why it is referred to as a fetus.

The most crucial time in the development of the baby is probably the first trimester. In the first two to three weeks of development, the spinal cord and neural plate (which eventually become the central nervous system) are formed. During the first three weeks of pregnancy, tissue that will later become the heart is already beginning to grow and take shape. In fact at the end of the first month of pregnancy, an S-shaped heart is beating on its own about 60 times per minute. Also by the end of the first month the three primary areas of the brain have already formed; small buds that will become the limbs are beginning to develop; the beginning of what will be the eyes and ears are visible; and the liver and blood vessels are forming.

During the second month of pregnancy, all major organs continue to grow and develop and the embryo becomes capable of movement. The major veins and arteries assume their final position in the embryo and the heart is now normally shaped and developed, albeit in miniature form. The brain is also beginning to send signals to the major organs to help regulate their function and a few minor reflexes are now evident. Also during the second month, the sex organs, bones, and muscles of the child have begun to form internally. By the end of the second month, all of the major organs are present, including the limbs and head, and the embryo looks like a little minature human being.

During the third month, the fetus begins breathing movements, which transfer amniotic fluid in and out of the lungs. Also, the eyes and ears are beginning to assume their final positions on the head and the arms and legs are very distinct. The fetus can carry on some sucking movements and the sex of the child is clearly identifiable. By the end of the third month, the fetus weights about 14 grams (½ ounce) and is about 56 millimeters (over 2 inches long).

During months 4 through 6, the fetus continues to grow and develop. The fetus is able to move independently throughout the amniotic sac and the heart is beating about 150 times a minute. At about the fifth month of pregnancy, the heartbeat can be heard using a stethoscope and the fetus is 250 millimeters (10 inches) in length, which is approximately half of its total length at birth.

The greatest amount of growth in the fetus occurs during the last trimester of pregnancy. The weight of the fetus will almost double during months 8 and 9. Also during this time, the final development of almost all the tissues and organs is taking place. The development of the ability of the fetus to regulate its own temperature and breathe air occurs during this part of the pregnancy.

Medication Use and Pregnancy

Most medical sources estimate the chances of a baby being born with a major birth defect at about 3 percent. Another 3 percent have birth defects that usually appear in the first year after birth. The cause of 40 percent of these birth defects is unknown. Another 12 to 25 percent of birth defects are caused by genetic defects in the infant or mother, of which Down syndrome is the most common. About 20 percent are due to interactions between hereditary factors and the environment. The causes of these are largely unknown. Finally, about 5 to 10 percent of all birth defects are the result of chemicals, drugs, and/or infections or diseases the mother has while pregnant. This may seem like a small percentage, but many of these are avoidable with proper education and counseling on drug therapy choices from the patient's doctor and pharmacist. It is important to know that almost every medication that a mother takes will reach the fetus. In fact, sometimes the fetus is receiving the same amount of drug as the mother via the umbilical cord. Therefore, pregnant women should think very carefully about the potential effects on the fetus before taking any medication.

There are two important factors that determine the potential harm to the fetus of a medication, length of exposure and age of the fetus at exposure. From fertilization to two weeks after fertilization, the embryo is relatively resistant to the effects of drugs. At this point in development, it is usually an "all or none response." The embryo will either survive from exposure to the drug or be unaffected. Major birth defects usually do not occur from drug exposure during this time.

Little is known regarding at which stage or trimester of pregnancy the fetus is at greatest risk for developing birth defects from medication use. However, weeks 2 through 10 appear to be a very critical time period. During this time, most of the major organs are forming and it may be when many birth defects occur. This is not to say, however, that medications taken during the second and third trimesters will not cause birth defects. Birth defects due to exposure to certain drugs can and do occur during the second and third trimesters, including central nervous system (CNS) development defects, growth problems, mental development disorders, reproductive defects, and many others. Finally, the longer a woman takes a drug the greater the risk of birth defects due to repeated exposure.

A definitive cause-and-effect relationship between a specific drug and birth defects can be hard to prove, because of many other factors and exposures a woman may experience during pregnancy. It's unethical to test the effects of medications on the fetus, so much of our information regarding the potential of drugs to cause birth defects comes from cases reported by physicians and from animal testing. Many medications are tested on pregnant rats, mice, and rabbits. These results may provide some useful insight into the potential effects in humans, but the true effect on the human fetus is still not known.

The Food and Drug Administration (FDA) instituted a ratings system for drugs marketed after 1980 based upon their perceived safety for use during pregnancy. The safest drugs are classified as Category A. These drugs have been shown to be of virtually no risk to the fetus and safe to take. Very, very few drugs are classified in Category A. Category X drugs, on the other hand, have been shown to definitely cause birth defects in the fetus when taken during pregnancy. The other categories—B, C, and D—fall somewhere in between categories A and X. A full explanation of each of the FDA categories of drug risk follows in Table 1.

TABLE 1: FDA CLASSIFICATION CATEGORIES OF FETAL RISK FROM DRUG THERAPY

CATEGORY A:

Controlled studies in women fail to demonstrate a risk to the fetus in the first trimester (and there is no evidence of a risk in later trimesters), and the possibility of fetal harm appears remote.

CATEGORY B:

1. Either animal-reproduction studies have not demonstrated a fetal risk but there are no controlled studies in pregnant women, or

2. animal-reproduction studies have shown an adverse effect that was not confirmed in controlled studies in women in the first trimester. Also, there is no evidence of a risk in later trimesters either.

CATEGORY C:

1. Studies in animals have revealed adverse effects on the fetus and there are no controlled studies in women, or

2. studies in women and animals are not available and the potential for adverse effects is unknown. These drugs should be given only if the potential benefits justify the potential risk to the fetus.

CATEGORY D:

There is positive evidence of human fetal risk, but the benefits from use in pregnant women may be acceptable despite the risk (e.g., if the drug is needed in a life-threatening situation or for a serious disease for which safer drugs cannot be used or are ineffective).

CATEGORY X:

Studies in animals or humans have demonstrated fetal abnormalities, there is evidence of fetal risk based on human experience, or both. The risk of the use of the drug in pregnant women clearly outweighs any possible benefits. The drug is contraindicated in women who are or may become pregnant.

Medication Use and Breast-feeding

Human milk is very complex and its exact chemical makeup is not known, but it does contain just the right amount of lactose, water, fatty acids, amino acids, and other components essential for the proper development of a young infant. Formula is similar to breast milk, but it is not a perfect match. Human milk contains at least 100 ingredients not found in formula. These ingredients include living cells, hormones, and active enzymes. Human milk also contains antibodies to disease and macrophages, cells that kill bacteria, fungi, and viruses. Therefore, when the mother is exposed to disease she makes antibodies to fight this disease. These antibodies are transferred to infants to help them fight off the disease as well. An infant's immune system will receive a great deal of help fighting infection and viruses. There is little doubt that breast milk is better for infants than formula.

Another benefit of breast milk is that it is always sterile when taken straight from the breast. Therefore, most common illnesses, such as colds, flu, skin infections, and diarrhea, cannot be passed from the mother to the infant through breast milk. The HIV virus, however, can be passed from mother to infant through breast milk. Much of what the mother eats and ingests is also found in breast milk. This includes many medications.

As a general rule, medications that are given to a mother reach the infant in much smaller quantities through her breast milk. However in some cases, even these smaller amounts can be harmful to the infant. When a breast-feeding mother takes a medication, her first response may be to stop breast-feeding altogether. This is not always best for the infant. A better goal is to minimize infant exposure to drugs in the breast milk, with minimal disruption in regular nursing patterns. The best alternative is to choose drugs that do not get into the breast milk or are known not to have adverse effects on the infant. But this is not always possible. Here are some tips, in order of importance, to follow when taking medication while breast-feeding.

1. Always talk to your doctor or pharmacist first.

2. Don't take the medication if it is not essential. For example: If you can suffer through the symptoms of a cold without taking medication, do it.

3. Choose drugs that do not get into the breast milk or are found in very low concentrations in breast milk. Your doctor or pharmacist can recommend these to you.

4. Wherever possible, use topically applied creams, ointment, nasal sprays, etc. The medications in these products are less likely to get into the breast milk.

5. Express or pump some milk from the breast and then take the medication. At the next feeding or two, use the milk that you have expressed or pumped.

6. Avoid nursing at times of peak drug concentration in milk. As a rule of thumb, peak concentration of a drug occurs in the milk about 1 to 3 hours after an oral dose. Therefore, nurse the infant just before you take a dose of medicine. This method works best for infants who nurse at regular 3- or 4-hour intervals rather than those still nursing every 2 hours or so.

7. Take the medication before the infant's longest sleep period. If the infant sleeps all night, take the medication after you put the infant down for the night.

8. Stop breast-feeding temporarily if you are taking the medication for a short time period and use formula instead. To maintain milk flow, it will be necessary to express or pump breast milk during this time. Just discard the expressed milk.

Each chapter in this book provides information regarding the risk to the infant of a particular drug, chemical, or toxin when breast-feeding. For many drugs, we do not currently know if they pass into breast milk or if they are a danger to the infant. Therefore, some entries state that researchers are unsure of the potential effects. In some instances, a drug may be safer to use during pregnancy than during breast-feeding. This could be because the drug is found in higher concentration in breast milk and potentially could do more harm to the infant.

The information within this book should only be used as a general guide to a broad spectrum of substances that can be harmful to the developing infant. Always consult your doctor or pharmacist regarding the safety of any medication, herb, vitamin supplement, or chemical and its potential effect on a breast-feeding infant.

OVERALL RECOMMENDATION: Before taking any prescription medication, over-the-counter drug, herbal or homeopathic product, vitamin, or the like, always consult your doctor or pharmacist first. If you can do without it, avoid it. Do not rely solely on the information from books, the Internet, friends, or family regarding the safe use of medication during pregnancy. Only a qualified doctor or pharmacist can provide this information.

CHAPTER 2

Prescription Drugs

Before marketing a new drug, the manufacturer almost never tests the product in pregnant women. Many drugs are not recommended for use during pregnancy due to a lack of information regarding their safety. Therefore, physicians must rely on case reports, animal testing, and their own personal experiences when deciding which medication is safe to prescribe for a patient who is pregnant. I've reviewed the current medical literature regarding the use in pregnancy of the top 200 prescription drugs taken by women ages 16 to 50.

Following is a listing of these prescription products in alphabetical order by brand name. Each entry will include the federal government's rating of risk. This is a rating the Food and Drug Administration (FDA) has assigned to the product based on its potential adverse effect on the fetus. For a discussion of this rating system, see pages 8–9 in Chapter 1. Next, a visual risk scale is provided to further illustrate the potential risk to the fetus. This scale was derived from the FDA rating and the medical literature that has documented potential risk to the fetus for specific products. The visual risk scale may indicate more risk in some instances than the FDA rating. The author considered other published studies and case reports when assigning a risk rating to each drug. Next, a short discussion of the potential adverse effects on the fetus is presented.

Each entry closes with a short discussion on the potential of the product to pass into the breast milk and cause adverse effects on a breast-feeding infant. Significantly less is known regarding which drugs are found in the breast milk, and potential effects of those drugs that do pass into the breast milk than the effects of these medications on the fetus. Therefore, some of these entries may seem ambiguous regarding their risk to a breast-feeding infant. Also, in some instances, a drug may be safer to use during pregnancy than during breast-feeding. This may be odd but is true. This could be because the drug is found in higher concentration in breast milk and potentially could do more harm to the infant. Finally, before taking any prescription drug during pregnancy, always consult your doctor or pharmacist first.

BRAND NAME: **Accolate**

GENERIC NAME: **zafirlukast**

USES: **To treat asthma and other breathing disorders**

FDA PREGNANCY CATEGORY: **B**

VIRTUALLY NO RISK	SLIGHT RISK	MODERATE RISK	STRONG RISK	EXTREME RISK

Accolate has not been studied in pregnant women. However, mice, rats, and monkeys were given doses up to 800 times the maximum daily dose for humans. At these high doses, no birth defects were found in these animals.

BREAST-FEEDING: This drug is found in breast milk and may be harmful to a breast-feeding infant. This drug should not be taken by nursing mothers.

BRAND NAME: **Accupril**

GENERIC NAME: **quinapril**

USES: **To treat high blood pressure and heart failure**

FDA PREGNANCY CATEGORY: **D**

VIRTUALLY NO RISK	SLIGHT RISK	MODERATE RISK	STRONG RISK	EXTREME RISK

Accupril should be used with extreme caution during pregnancy. In the second and third trimesters of pregnancy, this drug has been shown to cause severe birth defects and possible death of the fetus. During the first trimester of pregnancy, its safety is only slightly better. Therefore, this drug should not be used at all during pregnancy unless potential benefits strongly outweigh the very serious risks to the fetus.

BREAST-FEEDING: It is not known whether the drug is found in breast milk. Caution should be used when breast-feeding.

BRAND NAME: **Accutane**
GENERIC NAME: **isotretinoin**
USES: **To treat acne**
FDA PREGNANCY CATEGORY: **X**

VIRTUALLY NO RISK	SLIGHT RISK	MODERATE RISK	STRONG RISK	EXTREME RISK

Accutane is often used in young adults to treat severe acne. The drug is known to cause several serious birth defects in both humans and animals. The chance of a woman who is taking Accutane having a child with a major birth defect is greater than 20 percent, and the chance of having a miscarriage is about 18 percent. In fact, women who wish to become pregnant should stop taking the drug at least one month before trying to become pregnant. Under no circumstances should any woman ever take this drug who is pregnant or believes she may be pregnant.

BREAST-FEEDING: It is not known whether Accutane is excreted in the breast milk. Do not take this drug if breast-feeding due to possible health risks to the infant.

BRAND NAME: **Adalat CC**

GENERIC NAME: **nifedipine**

See entry for **Procardia XL**

BRAND NAME: **Aldomet**

GENERIC NAME: **methyldopa**

USES: **To treat high blood pressure**

FDA PREGNANCY CATEGORY: **C**

VIRTUALLY NO RISK	SLIGHT RISK	MODERATE RISK	STRONG RISK	EXTREME RISK
░░░░░	░░░░░	░░░░░		

This drug is known to cross the placenta. But studies have been conducted and have demonstrated that Aldomet is fairly safe for use during pregnancy. A mild reduction in infant blood pressure for the first two days after delivery has been noted, but the reduction is minimal.

BREAST-FEEDING: This drug is found in breast milk. However, the American Academy of Pediatrics considers it to be compatible with breast-feeding. However, some caution should still be used because of the potential to slightly lower the infant's blood pressure.

BRAND NAME: **Alesse-28**

GENERIC NAME: **levonorgestrel and ethinyl estradiol**

USES: **An oral contraceptive**

FDA PREGNANCY CATEGORY: **X**

VIRTUALLY NO RISK	SLIGHT RISK	MODERATE RISK	STRONG RISK	EXTREME RISK
░░░░░	░░░░░	░░░░░	░░░░░	░░░░░

With the use of this drug, an increased risk of physical malformations has been found in the fetus. An increase in the number of cardiovascular difficulties, spina bifida, Down syndrome, and eye and ear problems have also been reported with the use of hormones during pregnancy. Female fetuses exposed to the progesterone component have experienced some developmental changes, including masculinization. Exposure could also potentially cause developmental abnormalities of the sex organs in male babies, but is unlikely due to the low estrogen content of the product. Under no circumstances should any woman who is pregnant or believes she may be pregnant take this drug.

BREAST-FEEDING: This drug is found in breast milk. The potential effects of exposure to this drug on a breast-feeding infant are not known. Women taking this drug should use extreme caution when breast-feeding.

BRAND NAME: **Allegra**
GENERIC NAME: **fexofenadine**
USES: **To treat allergies**
FDA PREGNANCY CATEGORY: **C**

VIRTUALLY NO RISK	SLIGHT RISK	MODERATE RISK	STRONG RISK	EXTREME RISK

Allegra has been studied in rats and rabbits at high doses. No birth defects were detected. Adequate reports of this drug's effects in pregnant women are not available. This drug should be only be used during pregnancy if the benefit to the mother outweighs the unknown potential risks to the fetus.

BREAST-FEEDING: This drug is found in breast milk. The potential effects of exposure to this drug on a breast-feeding infant are not known. Women taking this drug should use caution when breast-feeding.

BRAND NAME: **Altace**

GENERIC NAME: **ramipril**

USES: **To treat high blood pressure and heart failure**

FDA PREGNANCY CATEGORY: **D**

VIRTUALLY NO RISK	SLIGHT RISK	MODERATE RISK	STRONG RISK	EXTREME RISK
▓	▓	▓		

Altace should be used with extreme caution during pregnancy. In the second and third trimesters of pregnancy, this drug has been shown to cause severe birth defects and possible death of the fetus. During the first trimester of pregnancy, its safety is only slightly better. Therefore, this drug should not be used at all during pregnancy unless your doctor determines with you that the potential benefits from taking the drug strongly outweigh the very serious risks to the fetus.

BREAST-FEEDING: It is not known whether the drug is found in breast milk. Caution should be used when breast-feeding.

BRAND NAME: **Amaryl**

GENERIC NAME: **glimepiride**

USES: **To treat diabetes**

FDA PREGNANCY CATEGORY: **C**

VIRTUALLY NO RISK	SLIGHT RISK	MODERATE RISK	STRONG RISK	EXTREME RISK
▓	▓	▓		

Amaryl is a drug used to control blood sugar in patients who have diabetes, and is usually not recommended for use during pregnancy. Although high blood glucose levels during pregnancy are associated with numerous types of birth defects, the use of Amaryl has also been related to death of the fetus in both rats and rabbits. There are no studies of Amaryl in pregnant women, so the drug is not recommended for use during pregnancy. Insulin is the drug of choice in pregnancy to control blood sugar in patients with diabetes.

BREAST-FEEDING: It is not known whether the drug is found in breast milk. Caution should be used when breast-feeding.

BRAND NAME: **Ambien**

GENERIC NAME: **zolpidem**

USES: **For short-term treatment of insomnia**

FDA PREGNANCY CATEGORY: **B**

VIRTUALLY NO RISK	SLIGHT RISK	MODERATE RISK	STRONG RISK	EXTREME RISK

There are no clinical studies regarding the use of Ambien during pregnancy. However, rats and rabbits were given this drug. Minimal defects were noted, but a decrease in fetal weight was observed. Because of the lack of reports in humans, other alternatives for insomnia may be preferred, such as relaxation therapy or possibly Benadryl.

BREAST-FEEDING: This drug is found in breast milk. The potential effects of exposure to this drug on a breast-feeding infant are not known. Nursing mothers taking this drug should use caution when breast-feeding.

BRAND NAME: **Amoxil**

GENERIC NAME: **amoxicillin**

USES: **To treat infections**

FDA PREGNANCY CATEGORY: **B**

VIRTUALLY NO RISK	SLIGHT RISK	MODERATE RISK	STRONG RISK	EXTREME RISK

Amoxil is a penicillin antibiotic. There have been no conclusive reports of birth defects caused by taking Amoxil in normal doses. Even doses as large as six 500mg capsules taken all at once by pregnant women have not been found to cause birth defects.

BREAST-FEEDING: This drug is found in breast milk. The American Academy of Pediatrics considers this drug to be compatible with breast-feeding. As with all drugs, some caution should still be used.

BRAND NAME: **Asacol**
GENERIC NAME: **mesalamine**
USES: **To treat mildly to moderately active ulcerative colitis**
FDA PREGNANCY CATEGORY: **B**

VIRTUALLY NO RISK	SLIGHT RISK	MODERATE RISK	STRONG RISK	EXTREME RISK

It is recommended that women who are on this drug and are in remission of ulcerative colitis should continue taking Asacol when trying to conceive or when pregnant to maintain remission. Only one instance of toxicity has been reported. It occurred when the mother was being treated with 4 grams per day between the thirteenth and twenty-fourth weeks of pregnancy. This report is controversial and no other birth defects have been noted. Overall, the benefits of this drug for the mother appear to outweigh the risks to the fetus.

BREAST-FEEDING: This drug is found in breast milk and may be harmful to a breast-feeding infant. This drug should not be taken by nursing mothers.

BRAND NAME: **Ativan**
GENERIC NAME: **lorazepam**
USES: **To treat anxiety and as sedation**
FDA PREGNANCY CATEGORY: **D**

VIRTUALLY NO RISK	SLIGHT RISK	MODERATE RISK	STRONG RISK	EXTREME RISK

No reports have been located linking Ativan to birth defects in humans. However, other drugs in the benzodiazepine family (Valium) have been suspected of causing fetal abnormalities such as cleft lip and palate and hernia. This drug does cross the placenta and can cause "floppy infant syndrome." Floppy infant syndrome occurs at birth and its symptoms include tiredness and sucking difficulties. When a mother takes high doses during pregnancy, her baby can suffer from withdrawal effects upon delivery, which include shakiness, diarrhea, vomiting, irritability, and slow growth. With these possible effects in mind, it is not advised to take Ativan during pregnancy.

BREAST-FEEDING: This drug is found in breast milk. The potential effects of exposure to this drug on a breast-feeding infant are not known. Nursing mothers taking this drug should use caution when breast-feeding.

BRAND NAME: **Atrovent**

GENERIC NAME: **ipratropium**

USES: **To treat bronchospasms associated with chronic obstructive pulmonary disease (COPD), including chronic bronchitis, emphysema, nasal allergies, and relief of nasal symptoms caused by the common cold.**

FDA PREGNANCY CATEGORY: **B**

VIRTUALLY NO RISK	SLIGHT RISK	MODERATE RISK	STRONG RISK	EXTREME RISK
▓▓▓▓▓▓	▓▓▓▓▓▓			

Atrovent is a compound used to open air passages in the lungs for treatment of asthmatic symptoms. Atrovent was not found to cause any birth defects in mice or rats when administered in doses of up to 2,000 times the maximum recommended oral human dose, or up to 312 times the maximum human dose for inhalation. Most sources suggest that inhaled Atrovent can safely be used in patients with severe asthma when other treatments have failed.

BREAST-FEEDING: It is not known whether the drug is found in breast milk. Caution should be used when breast-feeding.

BRAND NAME: **Augmentin**

GENERIC NAME: **Combination product containing amoxicillin and clavulanate potassium**

USES: **To treat bacterial infections**

FDA PREGNANCY CATEGORY: **B**

VIRTUALLY NO RISK	SLIGHT RISK	MODERATE RISK	STRONG RISK	EXTREME RISK

Augmentin has been studied in animals at very high doses of up to 200mg/kg/day. These high doses, which would be toxic in humans, showed no impairment of fertility or harm to the fetus. Only two small studies have been conducted in pregnant women who needed Augmentin for treatment of chlamydia, and results from these pregnancies were not reported. Augmentin should be used with some caution during pregnancy because of insufficient data proving its safety.

BREAST-FEEDING: This drug is found in breast milk. The potential effects of exposure to this drug on a breast-feeding infant are not known. Women taking this drug should use caution when breast-feeding.

BRAND NAME: **Avapro**

GENERIC NAME: **irbesartan**

USES: **To treat hypertension**

FDA PREGNANCY CATEGORY: **D**

VIRTUALLY NO RISK	SLIGHT RISK	MODERATE RISK	STRONG RISK	EXTREME RISK

Studies have not been reported using this drug in pregnant women. Avapro is assumed to cause birth defects due to its close relationship to drugs like Vasotec and Capoten. When used in the second and third trimesters, birth defects have been reported. Some of the effects include low blood pressure, kidney problems, anemia, and low red blood cell counts. Limb and facial deformities, lung development problems, stunted growth, and premature birth are all possible effects. Exposure during the first trimester may be safer, but extreme caution is needed if used during the second and third trimesters. With the risks associated with this drug, other treatment options, such as Aldomet, should be used first. This drug should be reserved for use as a last resort in treating high blood pressure.

BREAST-FEEDING: It is not known whether the drug is found in breast milk. Caution should be used when breast-feeding.

BRAND NAME: **Axid**
GENERIC NAME: **nizatidine**
USES: **For the treatment of active stomach ulcers, active duodenal ulcers (ulcers of the upper part of the small intestine, sometimes called peptic ulcers), maintenance of healed duodenal ulcers, and the treatment of gastroesophageal reflux disease (GERD)**
FDA PREGNANCY CATEGORY: **C**

VIRTUALLY NO RISK	SLIGHT RISK	MODERATE RISK	STRONG RISK	EXTREME RISK

Axid crosses the placenta. When given to pregnant rats and rabbits, no birth defects were reported in doses up to 1,500mg per kilogram of body weight. However, at the highest doses, abortions occurred in rabbits. Other birth defects, including spina bifida and an enlarged heart, were identified at lower doses in rabbits. With this information in mind, Axid should be used with caution during pregnancy.

BREAST-FEEDING: This drug is found in breast milk. The potential effects of exposure to this drug on a breast-feeding infant are not known. Women taking this drug should use caution when breast-feeding.

BRAND NAME: **Azmacort**

GENERIC NAME: **triamcinolone**

USES: **To treat asthma and other diseases causing inflammation in the lungs**

FDA PREGNANCY CATEGORY: **C**

VIRTUALLY NO RISK	SLIGHT RISK	MODERATE RISK	STRONG RISK	EXTREME RISK

Azmacort is a corticosteroid that is inhaled through the mouth and has shown to cause developmental abnormalities in animals. Birth defects such as cleft palate, growth retardation, hernias, altered male reproductive organs, and even fetal deaths have been shown in rats given this corticosteroid. Studies involving monkeys given intramuscular doses equal to and up to 300 times higher than normal human doses showed offspring with many birth defects, ranging from facial deformities to death. Azmacort should not be considered for use in pregnancy unless its benefits strongly outweigh the numerous risks involved.

BREAST-FEEDING: It is not known whether the drug is found in breast milk. Caution should be used when breast-feeding.

BRAND NAME: **Bactrim DS**

GENERIC NAME: **Combination product containing sulfamethoxazole and trimethoprim**

USES: **To treat bacterial infections**

FDA PREGNANCY CATEGORY: **C**

VIRTUALLY NO RISK	SLIGHT RISK	MODERATE RISK	STRONG RISK	EXTREME RISK

Bactrim DS is a combination antibiotic that contains two different ingredients, trimethoprim and sulfamethoxazole. Trimethoprim crosses the placenta and when studied in combination with sulfamethoxazole, has resulted in birth defects when administered to pregnant women. Sulfonamides, including sulfamethoxazole, are prescribed alone, or in combination with trimethoprim. Sulfonamides easily cross the placenta, and when given to females near delivery have resulted in severe jaundice (yellowing of the skin and eyes), anemia (decreased number of red blood cells), and kernicterus (toxicity in the brain caused by the jaundice). Sulfonamides should not be considered a treatment option for mothers who are at the end of their pregnancy. They are somewhat less dangerous when given at other times during pregnancy. Sulfonamides alone have been shown to cause developmental abnormalities in some animal species, although studies in humans have not proven a definite relationship between the drug and birth defects. In one study, a 5.5 percent incidence of birth defects resulted when patients were given the combination trimethoprim/sulfamethoxazole. Bactrim DS should be used with caution during pregnancy.

BREAST-FEEDING: This drug is found in breast milk. The American Academy of Pediatrics considers this drug to be compatible with breast-feeding. As with all drugs during pregnancy, some caution should still be used during breast-feeding.

BRAND NAME: **Bactroban**
GENERIC NAME: **mupirocin**
USES: **To treat bacterial skin infections and impetigo**
FDA PREGNANCY CATEGORY: **B**

VIRTUALLY NO RISK	SLIGHT RISK	MODERATE RISK	STRONG RISK	EXTREME RISK

Bactroban is a drug applied to the skin to treat various infections. In general, drugs that are applied topically are safer than those drugs taken by mouth. In rats and rabbits given oral and intramuscular doses up to 100 times the human topical dose, no harm to the fetus was reported. There are no studies on the use of Bactroban in humans, but the drug should be safe to use topically during pregnancy.

BREAST-FEEDING: It is not known whether the drug is found in breast milk, but it is unlikely to be found there. However, some caution should be used when breast-feeding.

BRAND NAME: **Beclovent**
GENERIC NAME: **beclomethasone dipropionate**
USES: **To treat asthma and other diseases causing inflammation in the lungs**
FDA PREGNANCY CATEGORY: **C**

VIRTUALLY NO RISK	SLIGHT RISK	MODERATE RISK	STRONG RISK	EXTREME RISK

Beclovent is an inhaled steroid used for the treatment of asthma and has been shown to cause birth defects in animals. Studies conducted in humans, however, could not prove a direct relationship between the drug's use and birth defects. In one study, exposure to the drug during the first trimester of pregnancy in 395 infants resulted in a 4.1 percent rate of birth defects. Specific information about these birth defects could not be obtained. Beclovent should only be used when its benefits strongly outweigh its possible risks to the fetus.

BREAST-FEEDING: It is not known whether the drug is found in breast milk. Caution should be used when breast-feeding.

BRAND NAME: **Bentyl**

GENERIC NAME: **dicyclomine**

USES: **To treat irritable bowel syndrome and other stomach and intestinal disorders**

FDA PREGNANCY CATEGORY: **C**

VIRTUALLY NO RISK	SLIGHT RISK	MODERATE RISK	STRONG RISK	EXTREME RISK

This drug has been used during pregnancy. In one study, minor malformations have been linked to use in the first trimester and include clubfoot, increased head size, and an increased number of fingers or toes. The authors of this study warned that a relationship could not be inferred from the data. Other studies could not specifically link birth defects to this drug. It appears that the use of Bentyl during pregnancy presents a moderate risk to the fetus.

BREAST-FEEDING: This drug is found in breast milk and may be harmful to a breast-feeding infant. This drug should not be taken by nursing mothers.

BRAND NAME: **Biaxin**

GENERIC NAME: **clarithromycin**

USES: **To treat bacterial infections**

FDA PREGNANCY CATEGORY: **C**

VIRTUALLY NO RISK	SLIGHT RISK	MODERATE RISK	STRONG RISK	EXTREME RISK

Biaxin, a derivative of erythromycin, is an antibiotic used to treat various bacterial infections. Studies in rats, mice, rabbits, and monkeys given doses of up to 160mg/kg/day (1.3 times the maximum recommended human dose), showed no harm to fertility or the fetus. At doses 2 to 4 times the maximum human dose, mice showed an increased number of offspring with cleft palate. Published reports concerning the use of Biaxin in humans are not available, but in various pregnant patients treated with Biaxin for upper respiratory infections, some birth defects were noticed. There have been several reports to the FDA concerning birth defects thought to be caused by Biaxin. However, there were many different problems reported, so a positive causal relationship between the drug and these birth defects cannot be established. Biaxin should not be used in pregnancy unless its potential benefits strongly outweigh its risks to the fetus.

BREAST-FEEDING: This drug is found in breast milk. The potential effects of exposure to this drug on a breast-feeding infant are not known. Nursing mothers taking this drug should use extreme caution when breast-feeding.

BRAND NAME: **Bumex**
GENERIC NAME: **bumetanide**
USES: **To treat fluid retention due to congestive heart failure, kidney disease, or cirrhosis of the liver; also used in controlling high blood pressure**
FDA PREGNANCY CATEGORY: **C**

VIRTUALLY NO RISK	SLIGHT RISK	MODERATE RISK	STRONG RISK	EXTREME RISK
▒	▒	▒		

Bumex is a diuretic (water pill) that has been shown to cause no developmental abnormalities in rats, mice, hamsters, or rabbits. No published reports regarding the use of Bumex in humans exist. However, a 5.1 percent incidence of major birth defects was observed in one study. Hypospadias, a birth defect where the opening to the penis is on the underside, has been associated with use of this class of drug. Although not recommended for use in pregnancy, very high blood pressure, congestive heart failure, and pulmonary edema are conditions where it may be used. Bumex should only be used in pregnancy when its benefits strongly outweigh the risks involved.

BREAST-FEEDING: It is not known whether the drug is found in breast milk. Caution should be used when breast-feeding.

BRAND NAME: **BuSpar**
GENERIC NAME: **buspirone**
USES: **To treat anxiety**
FDA PREGNANCY CATEGORY: **B**

VIRTUALLY NO RISK	SLIGHT RISK	MODERATE RISK	STRONG RISK	EXTREME RISK
▨	▨			

This drug has shown minimal risks when used during pregnancy. In rats and rabbits, doses up to 30 times the maximum human dose have been administered. At these high doses, no adverse fetal effects were found.

BREAST-FEEDING: This drug is found in breast milk. The potential effects of exposure to this drug on a breast-feeding infant are not known. Nursing mothers taking this drug should use caution when breast-feeding.

BRAND NAME: **Calan**
GENERIC NAME: **verapamil**
USES: **To treat angina and high blood pressure**
FDA PREGNANCY CATEGORY: **C**

VIRTUALLY NO RISK	SLIGHT RISK	MODERATE RISK	STRONG RISK	EXTREME RISK
▨	▨			

This drug crosses the placenta. This drug can be given to mothers to treat heart conditions in the fetus. One study found no increase in the risk of malformations when this drug was given. This drug has even been administered during the first trimester without major fetal problems. Low blood pressure and a decrease in oxygen to the fetus do remain a risk. Calan should be used with some caution during pregnancy.

BREAST-FEEDING: This drug is found in breast milk. The American Academy of Pediatrics considers this drug to be compatible with breast-feeding. As with all drugs, caution should still be used.

BRAND NAME: **Capoten**
GENERIC NAME: **captopril**
Very similar to **Accupril;** see entry for **Accupril**

BRAND NAME: **Carafate**
GENERIC NAME: **sucralfate**
USES: **The treatment and prevention of ulcers**
FDA PREGNANCY CATEGORY: **B**

VIRTUALLY NO RISK	SLIGHT RISK	MODERATE RISK	STRONG RISK	EXTREME RISK

Carafate is an aluminum salt that is used to coat the stomach and protect against ulcers. In animal studies, doses up to 50 times the normal human dose showed no resulting birth defects. The possible toxicity from this drug comes from the aluminum, which may cause problems in the development of the brain and bones of the fetus. The actual absorption of the aluminum from the stomach is usually less than 15 percent. Due to this small amount of aluminum absorption, Carafate is considered an agent that may be used in pregnancy because its benefits currently outweigh its risks to the fetus.

BREAST-FEEDING: This drug is not found in breast milk; therefore women may breast-feed while taking this drug.

BRAND NAME: **Cardene**

GENERIC NAME: **nicardipine**

USES: **To treat angina and high blood pressure**

FDA PREGNANCY CATEGORY: **C**

VIRTUALLY NO RISK	SLIGHT RISK	MODERATE RISK	STRONG RISK	EXTREME RISK

Cardene does not appear to cause birth defects in rats and rabbits. It has been used in treating pregnant women, and passage of this drug to the placenta occurred in some cases, but no adverse effects were found in this study. This drug has been examined during different trimesters and appears to pose no increased risk of birth defects. However, some caution should still be used.

BREAST-FEEDING: This drug is found in breast milk. The potential effects of exposure to this drug on a breast-feeding infant are not known. Nursing mothers taking this drug should use caution when breast-feeding.

BRAND NAME: **Cardizem, Cardizem CD, and Cardizem SR**

GENERIC NAME: **diltiazem**

USES: **To treat angina and high blood pressure**

FDA PREGNANCY CATEGORY: **C**

VIRTUALLY NO RISK	SLIGHT RISK	MODERATE RISK	STRONG RISK	EXTREME RISK

Cardizem has been given to mice, rats, and rabbits in doses of 5 to 10 times the human daily dose. At these high doses, increased mortality and birth defects have occurred in the animals. When this drug is given to pregnant women, minimal defects were noted but could not be causally linked to this drug. Most reports of the use of this drug during pregnancy found no major risk of birth defects. However, because of the chance of defects, this drug should be used with caution during pregnancy.

BREAST-FEEDING: This drug is found in breast milk. The potential effects of exposure to this drug on a breast-feeding infant are not known. Nursing mothers taking this drug should use caution when breast-feeding.

BRAND NAME: **Cardura**
GENERIC NAME: **doxazosin**
USES: **To treat high blood pressure**
FDA PREGNANCY CATEGORY: **C**

VIRTUALLY NO RISK	SLIGHT RISK	MODERATE RISK	STRONG RISK	EXTREME RISK

Cardura is a drug used to treat high blood pressure. In pregnant rats and rabbits given doses 75 and 150 times the maximum recommended human daily dose, respectively, no effects on the fetus were seen. Slowed growth after delivery was observed in rat pups after Cardura was given during pregnancy. No studies of the use of Cardura in humans during pregnancy exist. This drug should not be used in pregnancy unless its benefits clearly outweigh its potential risks to the fetus.

BREAST-FEEDING: This drug is found in breast milk. The potential effects of exposure to this drug on a breast-feeding infant are not known. Nursing mothers taking this drug should use caution when breast-feeding.

BRAND NAME: **Ceclor**
GENERIC NAME: **cefaclor**
USES: **To treat bacterial infections**
FDA PREGNANCY CATEGORY: **B**

VIRTUALLY NO RISK	SLIGHT RISK	MODERATE RISK	STRONG RISK	EXTREME RISK

Ceclor is an oral antibiotic that is usually considered safe for use during pregnancy. Studies conducted in mice, rats, and ferrets found no harmful effects on fertility or to the fetus at doses up to 12 times the normal human dose. In one study, Ceclor exposure during the first trimester was analyzed and 5.7 percent of the newborns had birth defects, including cardiovascular defects, spina bifida, and defects within their limbs. It is proposed that some of the mother's disease states and the use of other drugs could have contributed to these birth defects as well.

BREAST-FEEDING: This drug is found in breast milk. The potential effects of exposure to this drug on a breast-feeding infant are not known. Nursing mothers taking this drug should use caution when breast-feeding.

BRAND NAME: **Cedax**
GENERIC NAME: **ceftibuten**
USES: **To treat bacterial infections**
FDA PREGNANCY CATEGORY: **B**

VIRTUALLY NO RISK	SLIGHT RISK	MODERATE RISK	STRONG RISK	EXTREME RISK

Cedax is an oral antibiotic used to treat bacterial infections, and is usually considered safe for use in pregnancy. Studies in rats showed no harm to fertility in doses up to 43 times the recommended human dose. No harm to the fetus was observed in rat studies at doses up to 8.6 times the recommended human dose. No reports concerning the use of Cedax in human pregnancy are available.

BREAST-FEEDING: It is not known whether the drug is found in breast milk. Caution should be used when breast-feeding.

BRAND NAME: **Ceftin**

GENERIC NAME: **cefuroxime**

USES: **To treat bacterial infections**

FDA PREGNANCY CATEGORY: **B**

VIRTUALLY NO RISK	SLIGHT RISK	MODERATE RISK	STRONG RISK	EXTREME RISK

Ceftin is an oral antibiotic that is usually considered safe for use during pregnancy. Studies in mice and rats showed no harm to the fetus in doses up to 23 times the maximum recommended human dose. In one large study involving humans, a very small percentage of birth defects was observed in patients who had received Ceftin during the first trimester. However, this study could not prove a relationship between taking the drug and the birth defects.

BREAST-FEEDING: This drug is found in breast milk. The potential effects of exposure to this drug on a breast-feeding infant are not known. Nursing mothers taking this drug should use caution when breast-feeding.

BRAND NAME: **Cefzil**

GENERIC NAME: **cefprozil**

USES: **To treat bacterial infections**

FDA PREGNANCY CATEGORY: **B**

VIRTUALLY NO RISK	SLIGHT RISK	MODERATE RISK	STRONG RISK	EXTREME RISK

Cefzil is an oral anti-infective and is usually considered safe for use during pregnancy. Although no reports concerning the use of Cefzil in pregnancy are available, reproductive studies in mice found no harm to the fetus at doses up to 14 times the maximum recommended daily human dose. In studies conducted in rats and rabbits, doses up to 7 and 14 times the maximum recommended human dose showed no harm to the fetus.

BREAST-FEEDING: This drug is found in breast milk. The American Academy of Pediatrics considers this drug to be compatible with breast-feeding. As with all drugs, some caution should still be taken.

BRAND NAME: **Celebrex**
GENERIC NAME: **celecoxib**
USES: **Osteoarthritis and adult rheumatoid arthritis**
FDA PREGNANCY CATEGORY: **C**

VIRTUALLY NO RISK	SLIGHT RISK	MODERATE RISK	STRONG RISK	EXTREME RISK

There are no clinical studies regarding the use of Celebrex during pregnancy. However, in rats at high doses, fused ribs and hernias were noted. Also, problems with egg implantation may arise due to the way the drug works. If used in the third trimester, the fetus's heart may not form correctly. This drug should only be used during pregnancy if its potential benefit outweighs the risk of harm to the fetus.

BREAST-FEEDING: It is not known whether the drug is found in breast milk. Caution should be used when breast-feeding.

BRAND NAME: **Celexa**
GENERIC NAME: **citalopram**
USES: **To treat depression**
FDA PREGNANCY CATEGORY: **C**

VIRTUALLY NO RISK	SLIGHT RISK	MODERATE RISK	STRONG RISK	EXTREME RISK

Limited studies have been done using Celexa during pregnancy. It was found that when this drug is used, there is an increased risk of birth defects, mainly heart and skeletal defects. Other drugs in the selective serotonin reuptake inhibitor (SSRI) family have shown some minor malformations, including heart malformations. There is also an increased risk of decreased birth weight, complications with breathing, and death to the fetus. With no concrete evidence of this drug causing major birth defects, doctors generally prefer to use Prozac over Celexa if there is a need to treat serious episodes of depression.

BREAST-FEEDING: This drug is found in breast milk. The potential effects of exposure to this drug on a breast-feeding infant are not known. Nursing mothers taking this drug should use caution when breast-feeding.

BRAND NAME: **Cipro**
GENERIC NAME: **ciprofloxacin**
USES: **To treat bacterial infections**
FDA PREGNANCY CATEGORY: **C**

VIRTUALLY NO RISK	SLIGHT RISK	MODERATE RISK	STRONG RISK	EXTREME RISK

Cipro is a antibiotic that is generally not recommended for use during pregnancy. Several studies have been conducted in women. Birth defects, including developmental retardation, discoloration of the teeth, low birth weight, and even miscarriage, have been reported. Studies have also shown damage to the cartilage in various joints in immature rats and dogs, and some joint abnormalities have been noted in children exposed to Cipro during pregnancy. Although these results do not establish a definite relationship between drug exposure and birth defects, Cipro should absolutely not be taken during the first trimester because of the abnormalities observed in animals when exposed to Cipro during this time. Cipro should be avoided throughout the rest of pregnancy as well.

BREAST-FEEDING: This drug is found in breast milk and may be harmful to a breast-feeding infant. This drug should not be taken by nursing mothers.

BRAND NAME: **Claritin**

GENERIC NAME: **loratadine**

USES: **To treat allergies**

FDA PREGNANCY CATEGORY: **B**

VIRTUALLY NO RISK	SLIGHT RISK	MODERATE RISK	STRONG RISK	EXTREME RISK

There are no clinical studies regarding the use of Claritin during pregnancy. Six reports of birth defects have been identified, including cleft palate and deafness. However, a definite relationship between this drug and these events cannot be determined. In rats and rabbits, greater than 75 to 150 times the dose was given. At these high doses, no birth defects were noted in these animals. This drug should be used with some caution during pregnancy because potential adverse effects on the fetus have not been studied.

BREAST-FEEDING: This drug is found in breast milk. The potential effects of exposure to this drug on a breast-feeding infant are not known. Nursing mothers taking this drug should use caution when breast-feeding.

BRAND NAME: **Cleocin T**

GENERIC NAME: **clindamycin**

USES: **To treat acne and vaginal bacterial infections**

FDA PREGNANCY CATEGORY: **B**

VIRTUALLY NO RISK	SLIGHT RISK	MODERATE RISK	STRONG RISK	EXTREME RISK

Cleocin T is a topical antibiotic solution used to treat various bacterial infections. In general, drugs applied topically are safer than those drugs taken by mouth. No reports are available to establish a definite relationship between clindamycin and birth defects. Oral clindamycin easily crosses the placenta, and has been used in women to prevent infection before a cesarean section is performed. In a Michigan study, 647 infants had been exposed to clindamycin, either taken orally or used topically, during the first trimester and 4.8 percent of these infants had major birth defects. This small percentage does not provide a definite relationship between the drug and these birth defects in the fetus.

BREAST-FEEDING: This drug is found in breast milk. The American Academy of Pediatrics considers this drug to be compatible with breast-feeding. As with all drugs, though, some caution should still be used.

BRAND NAME: **Clinoril**
GENERIC NAME: **sulindac**
USES: **To treat arthritis, gouty arthritis, and for pain relief**
FDA PREGNANCY CATEGORY: **B**

VIRTUALLY NO RISK	SLIGHT RISK	MODERATE RISK	STRONG RISK	EXTREME RISK

Clinoril is a nonsteroidal anti-inflammatory drug (NSAID) used to treat pain and arthritis. When given to pregnant rats, Clinoril caused a decrease in fetal weight, made the pregnancy longer, and caused problems with labor and delivery. Women who are trying to conceive should not take Clinoril because it may block the implantation of the fertilized egg. Clinoril should not be given in the third trimester or near delivery because it may inhibit the natural labor process, cause high blood pressure in the lungs of the fetus, and decrease the kidney function of the fetus. Clinoril also has been shown to decrease the amount of fluid produced by the fetus.

BREAST-FEEDING: It is not known whether the drug is found in breast milk. Caution should be used when breast-feeding.

BRAND NAME: **Coumadin**

GENERIC NAME: **warfarin**

USES: **To treat thromboembolic disorders; it is an anticoagulant**

FDA PREGNANCY CATEGORY: **X**

VIRTUALLY NO RISK	SLIGHT RISK	MODERATE RISK	STRONG RISK	EXTREME RISK

Coumadin is known to cause several serious birth defects in both humans and animals. Central nervous system problems, miscarriage, bleeding, premature birth and stillbirth have all been reported. Fetal warfarin syndrome has also been reported and includes nose flattening, respiratory problems, deafness, seizures, and death. Lower IQs have been found in children following exposure to this drug. In most cases, the chance of a woman on Coumadin having a normal child is less than 70 percent. Under no circumstances should any woman who is pregnant take this drug.

BREAST-FEEDING: This drug is found in breast milk. The potential effects of exposure to this drug on a breast-feeding infant are not known, but could be dangerous. Because this drug can cause serious birth defects in the fetus, nursing mothers taking this drug should use extreme caution when breast-feeding.

BRAND NAME: **Cozaar**

GENERIC NAME: **losartan**

USES: **To treat high blood pressure**

FDA PREGNANCY CATEGORY: **D**

VIRTUALLY NO RISK	SLIGHT RISK	MODERATE RISK	STRONG RISK	EXTREME RISK

Cozaar is believed to cause birth defects because of its close chemical relationship to drugs such as Vasotec and Capoten, which are known to do so. When Cozaar is used in the second and third trimesters, birth defects have been reported. Among these are low blood pressure, renal problems, anemia, and low red blood cell counts. Limb and facial deformities are also a possibility, along with lung development problems. A possibility exists for stunted growth and premature birth. Exposure during the first trimester may be safer, but extreme caution is needed during the second and third trimesters. With the risks associated with this drug, other treatment options should be used first. This drug should be reserved as a last resort in treating high blood pressure.

BREAST-FEEDING: It is not known whether the drug is found in breast milk. Caution should be used when breast-feeding.

BRAND NAME: **Darvocet N**
GENERIC NAME: **Combination product containing acetaminophen and propoxyphene**
USES: **To treat mild to moderate pain**
FDA PREGNANCY CATEGORY: **C**

VIRTUALLY NO RISK	SLIGHT RISK	MODERATE RISK	STRONG RISK	EXTREME RISK
▨	▨	▨		

Four case reports of use during pregnancy have noted infant abnormalities. Withdrawal has also been noted in five infants when their mothers ingested large amounts of this drug. This drug should be used with caution. If used for prolonged periods, the risk of birth defects increases significantly.

BREAST-FEEDING: This drug is found in breast milk. The potential effects of exposure to this drug on a breast-feeding infant are not known. Nursing mothers taking this drug should use extreme caution when breast-feeding.

BRAND NAME: **Daypro**

GENERIC NAME: **oxaprozin**

USES: **To treat arthritis and provide pain relief**

FDA PREGNANCY CATEGORY: **C**

VIRTUALLY NO RISK	SLIGHT RISK	MODERATE RISK	STRONG RISK	EXTREME RISK

There are no clinical studies regarding the use of Daypro during pregnancy. In animal studies, fetal abnormalities have been minimal. When Daypro is used in the third trimester, abnormally high blood pressure has been found in the lungs of the infants. Also, this agent should be avoided in those trying to conceive because the drug can block implantation of the egg. When used near delivery or in the third trimester, this drug is classified as a strong risk because of the possible increase in blood pressure in the fetal lungs. This drug has also been shown to prolong pregnancies and inhibit labor. This drug should be used with extreme caution during pregnancy, especially in the third trimester.

BREAST-FEEDING: It is not known whether the drug is found in breast milk. Caution should be used when breast-feeding.

BRAND NAME: **Deconsal II**

GENERIC NAME: **Combination product containing pseudoephedrine and guaifenesin**

USES: **To treat nasal congestion and cough**

FDA PREGNANCY CATEGORY: **C**

VIRTUALLY NO RISK	SLIGHT RISK	MODERATE RISK	STRONG RISK	EXTREME RISK

Deconsal II is a drug that contains two ingredients—pseudoephedrine and guaifenesin. Pseudoephedrine, and other drugs in this category, has been shown to cause birth defects in animals. Human studies in which first-trimester exposure to pseudoephedrine is reported have shown a significantly increased risk of fetal malformations. Many physicians suggest avoiding pseudoephedrine during the first trimester and using some caution during the second and third trimesters. One report of an infant who was exposed to both pseudoephedrine and guaifenesin during pregnancy showed some signs similar to fetal alcohol syndrome. Deconosal II is not recommended for use in pregnancy unless its benefits outweigh its risks to the fetus.

BREAST-FEEDING: It is not known whether the drug is found in breast milk. Caution should be used when breast-feeding.

BRAND NAME: **Depakote**

GENERIC NAME: **divalproex sodium (valproic acid)**

USES: **To manage seizures, mania, and help prevent migraine headaches**

FDA PREGNANCY CATEGORY: **D**

VIRTUALLY NO RISK	SLIGHT RISK	MODERATE RISK	STRONG RISK	EXTREME RISK

Depakote is a drug used to prevent seizures and is generally not considered a drug of choice in pregnant women. The use of Depakote during pregnancy has produced almost every kind of birth defect, with neural tube defects being the most common. Other birth defects linked to the use of Depakote include abnormal anatomy of the heart and blood vessels, facial and skeletal deformities, skin/muscle deformities, and mental retardation. In an observational study, 19.2 percent of the 26 newborns exposed to Depakote during the first trimester had some sort of major birth defect. Other problems associated with the use of Depakote by the mother include liver toxicity in the fetus and fetal distress during labor. The use of Depakote is not recommended during pregnancy. However, note that an epileptic mother has a two to three times greater chance of having a child with some kind of birth defect without any drug treatment. The use of Depakote should only be considered if the potential benefits very strongly outweigh the high possibility of birth defects in the fetus.

BREAST-FEEDING: This drug is found in breast milk and may be harmful to a breast-feeding infant. This drug should not be taken by nursing mothers.

BRAND NAME: **Desyrel**
GENERIC NAME: **trazodone**
USES: **To treat depression and insomnia**
FDA PREGNANCY CATEGORY: **C**

VIRTUALLY NO RISK	SLIGHT RISK	MODERATE RISK	STRONG RISK	EXTREME RISK

There are no clinical studies regarding the use of Desyrel during pregnancy. At high doses in animals, this drug is toxic and causes birth defects. Early termination of pregnancy has occurred, but no definite link can be made to this drug. Others drugs, such as Prozac, are probably a better choice to treat depression during pregnancy.

BREAST-FEEDING: This drug is found in breast milk and may be harmful to a breast-feeding infant. This drug should not be taken by nursing mothers.

BRAND NAME: **DiaBeta**
GENERIC NAME: **glyburide**
USES: **To treat diabetes**
FDA PREGNANCY CATEGORY: **B**

VIRTUALLY NO RISK	SLIGHT RISK	MODERATE RISK	STRONG RISK	EXTREME RISK

DiaBeta is an oral agent used to control the blood sugar of patients with type II diabetes and is not considered the drug of choice in pregnant diabetics. In studies conducted with pregnant mothers who received various medications (including DiaBeta) to control their blood sugar, a large percentage of the infants showed one or more malformations. These malformations included deformities of the face, heart, and central nervous system. Although a high percentage of birth defects resulted from the mothers who took the drugs, researchers also believe that poor control of the mother's blood sugar also could have contributed to these birth defects. DiaBeta should not be prescribed for pregnant diabetic patients. Insulin should be used to control blood sugar levels in these patients.

BREAST-FEEDING: It is not known whether the drug is found in breast milk. Caution should be used when breast-feeding.

BRAND NAME: **Diflucan**
GENERIC NAME: **fluconazole**
USES: **For treatment of vaginal candidiasis**
FDA PREGNANCY CATEGORY: **C**

VIRTUALLY NO RISK	SLIGHT RISK	MODERATE RISK	STRONG RISK	EXTREME RISK

Data regarding the use of this drug during pregnancy is very limited. At high doses, abortions and structural defects such as cleft palate have occurred in rats and rabbits. When doses of 400mg per day or more are used in the first trimester, this drug has caused fetal abnormalities in head and facial structures, bone formation, and heart development. Its safety at lower doses has not been identified, but appears low risk for short, low-dose therapy for vaginal fungal infections. This medication should be used with caution and at low doses during pregnancy.

BREAST-FEEDING: It is not known whether the drug is found in breast milk. Caution should be used when breast-feeding.

BRAND NAME: **Dilantin**

GENERIC NAME: **phenytoin**

USES: **Antiepileptic drug to control seizures**

FDA PREGNANCY CATEGORY: **D**

VIRTUALLY NO RISK	SLIGHT RISK	MODERATE RISK	STRONG RISK	EXTREME RISK

Dilantin is a drug used to prevent seizures in epileptic patients. The adverse effects of the drug during pregnancy are widely studied and proven. Women taking Dilantin are 2 to 3 times more likely to have children with birth defects when compared to the normal pregnant population. It is not known whether the disease, the drugs, or genetic factors play a major role in causing these defects. Almost all types of birth defects have been reported in children who have been exposed to Dilantin during pregnancy, as well as an increased risk for bleeding in the newborn after delivery. The use of Dilantin during pregnancy carries with it a significant risk for causing birth defects in the fetus. However, a risk–benefit ratio must be analyzed to determine if the potential benefit of controlling the seizures outweighs the potential for very serious birth defects. If Dilantin is used during the pregnancy, blood levels of the drug should be monitored often and kept at the lowest possible level to prevent seizures.

BREAST-FEEDING: This drug is found in breast milk. The potential effects of exposure to this drug on a breast-feeding infant are not known. Nursing mothers taking this drug should use extreme caution when breast-feeding.

BRAND NAME: **Diovan**

GENERIC NAME: **valsartan**

Similar to **Cozaar;** see entry for **Cozaar**

BRAND NAME: **Duricef**

GENERIC NAME: **cefadroxil**

USES: **To treat bacterial infections**

FDA PREGNANCY CATEGORY: **B**

VIRTUALLY NO RISK	SLIGHT RISK	MODERATE RISK	STRONG RISK	EXTREME RISK

Duricef is an antibiotic that is usually considered safe for use during pregnancy. Studies conducted on mice and rats found no adverse effects on fertility or harm to the fetus in doses up to 11 times the normal human dose. In one study of pregnant women, Duricef exposure during the first trimester showed a small percentage of major birth defects, including cardiovascular problems, spina bifida, and defects in the arms/legs. This data does not prove that Duricef was the cause of these birth defects. They could have resulted from factors that did not involve taking the drug, such as the mother's health and exposure to other harmful substances.

BREAST-FEEDING: This drug is found in breast milk. The American Academy of Pediatrics considers this drug to be compatible with breast-feeding. As with all drugs, some caution should still be used.

BRAND NAME: **Dyazide**

GENERIC NAME: **Combination product containing triamterene and hydrochlorothiazide**

USES: **To correct fluid retention (edema) seen in congestive heart failure and kidney or liver disease, and to treat high blood pressure**

FDA PREGNANCY CATEGORY: **C**

VIRTUALLY NO RISK	SLIGHT RISK	MODERATE RISK	STRONG RISK	EXTREME RISK
░	░	░		

This combination product should be avoided during the first trimester because of an increased risk of birth defects, among them heart and structural problems. This drug may also decrease blood to the placenta and increase the blood sugar of the mother. This could cause the baby to suffer from low blood sugar at birth. The use of this drug later in pregnancy may hold less risk. Dyazide may also slow down labor. Use of this drug should be avoided unless there are no other options for patients with heart disease.

BREAST-FEEDING: This drug is found in breast milk. The potential effects of exposure to this drug on a breast-feeding infant are not known. Nursing mothers taking this drug should use some caution when breast-feeding.

BRAND NAME: **DynaCirc**

GENERIC NAME: **isradipine**

USES: **To treat high blood pressure**

FDA PREGNANCY CATEGORY: **C**

VIRTUALLY NO RISK	SLIGHT RISK	MODERATE RISK	STRONG RISK	EXTREME RISK
░	░	░		

This drug does not cause birth defects in rats or rabbits at high doses. In human studies, no major adverse effects were noted, except low birth weight in one infant and jaundice in two others. However, due to the lack of clinical studies in humans, the drug should be used with caution.

BREAST-FEEDING: This drug is found in breast milk. The potential effects of exposure to this drug on a breast-feeding infant are not known. Nursing mothers taking this drug should use caution when breast-feeding.

BRAND NAME: **Effexor**
GENERIC NAME: **venlafaxine**
USES: **To treat depression**
FDA PREGNANCY CATEGORY: **C**

VIRTUALLY NO RISK	SLIGHT RISK	MODERATE RISK	STRONG RISK	EXTREME RISK

Effexor is a drug used primarily to treat depression. Studies conducted in rabbits with doses up to 12 times the maximum recommended human dose showed no developmental abnormalities. However, when rats were given up to 10 times the maximum recommended human dose throughout pregnancy and weaning, newborn weight was decreased and there was an increased rate of stillbirth and death during lactation. In a review of 10 women who used Effexor for a period of 10 to 60 days during their first trimester, no birth defects were observed in 4 of the infants, and no other information was provided for the other pregnancies. Effexor should be used with caution during pregnancy due to the lack of safety data.

BREAST-FEEDING: It is not known whether the drug is found in breast milk. Caution should be used when breast-feeding.

BRAND NAME: **Elavil**

GENERIC NAME: **amitriptyline**

USES: **To treat depression and insomnia**

FDA PREGNANCY CATEGORY: **D**

VIRTUALLY NO RISK	SLIGHT RISK	MODERATE RISK	STRONG RISK	EXTREME RISK

Fetal abnormalities have resulted from the use of this drug by pregnant mothers. One infant was born with cleft palate, foot deformations, and a lack of genital formation following a mother's overdose. Withdrawal has been a problem with other drugs used for depression, so the potential exists for this complication as well. This drug should only be used if its benefits significantly outweigh its risks.

BREAST-FEEDING: This drug is found in breast milk and may be harmful to a breast-feeding infant. This drug should not be taken by nursing mothers.

BRAND NAME: **Elocon**

GENERIC NAME: **mometasone**

USES: **To treat skin rashes, swelling, and itching**

FDA PREGNANCY CATEGORY: **C**

VIRTUALLY NO RISK	SLIGHT RISK	MODERATE RISK	STRONG RISK	EXTREME RISK

Elocon is a topical corticosteroid that is generally not recommended for use in pregnancy. In rats treated with topical doses up to 4 times the maximum recommended human dose, hernias, underdeveloped bones, and abnormal ribs were observed in the offspring. There are no studies of the effects of Elocon in pregnant women, so it should not be used in pregnancy unless its benefits outweigh its risks to the fetus.

BREAST-FEEDING: It is not known whether the drug is found in breast milk. Caution should be used when breast-feeding.

BRAND NAME: **E-Mycin**

GENERIC NAME: **erythromycin**

USES: **To treat bacterial infections**

FDA PREGNANCY CATEGORY: **B**

VIRTUALLY NO RISK	SLIGHT RISK	MODERATE RISK	STRONG RISK	EXTREME RISK
▨				

Erythromycin is an antibiotic used to treat various bacterial infections. No data is available that makes a definite connection between the use of erythromycin and birth defects. In one large study, 230 pregnant women took erythromycin at some point during the pregnancy. No direct evidence was found that linked the drug to any type of birth defect. The drug is generally considered safe to use for short periods of time during pregnancy.

BREAST-FEEDING: This drug is found in breast milk. The potential effects of exposure to this drug on a breast-feeding infant are not known. Nursing mothers taking this drug should use some caution when breast-feeding.

BRAND NAME: **Entex**

GENERIC NAME: **Combination product containing various combinations of phenylephrine, pseudoephedrine, and guaifenesin**

USES: **To treat nasal congestion and cough**

FDA PREGNANCY CATEGORY: **C**

VIRTUALLY NO RISK	SLIGHT RISK	MODERATE RISK	STRONG RISK	EXTREME RISK
▨	▨	▨		

This combination medicine has a potential risk of such infant birth defects as eye and ear problems, a depressed sternum, and clubfoot. There is an association of the phenylephrine component of this drug with an increased risk of birth defects. This drug is not recommended for pregnant women because other options exist that have fewer risks to the fetus.

BREAST-FEEDING: This drug is found in breast milk. The potential effects of exposure to this drug on a breast-feeding infant are not known. Nursing mothers taking this drug should use caution when breast-feeding.

BRAND NAME: **Ery-Tab**
GENERIC NAME: **erythromycin base**
See entry for **E-Mycin**

BRAND NAME: **Esgic**
GENERIC NAME: **Combination product containing acetaminophen, butalbital, and caffeine**
See entry for **Fioricet**

BRAND NAME: **Fioricet**
GENERIC NAME: **Combination product containing acetaminophen, butalbital, and caffeine**
USES: **To treat tension headache and for pain relief**
FDA PREGNANCY CATEGORY: **C**

VIRTUALLY NO RISK	SLIGHT RISK	MODERATE RISK	STRONG RISK	EXTREME RISK

Fioricet is a combination of three ingredients—butalbital, acetaminophen, and caffeine. When used in small amounts, caffeine has not been associated with malformations or miscarriages. High doses of caffeine may be responsible for miscarriage, difficulty in becoming pregnant, and infertility. Increased heart rate and breathing rate have been observed in a fetus who has been exposed to high amounts of caffeine. Butalbital is a barbiturate drug usually used to treat pain. In 112 newborns exposed to butalbital during the first trimester, there were no malformations reported. No adequate studies have been conducted in animals to determine if butalbital causes birth defects. In one human study, a small percentage of birth defects, including cardiovascular problems and spina bifida, were reported. Butalbital should not be considered for long-term use or in high doses near the end of pregnancy because of the potential to cause withdrawal symptoms in newborns. Acetaminophen (Tylenol®) is generally considered safe for use during all trimesters of pregnancy for short-term pain relief and fever reduction. Unlike aspirin, acetaminophen does not interfere with platelet function and therefore does not cause a problem with bleeding when given near delivery. This combination product is not recommended during pregnancy unless its potential benefits outweigh the risks involved.

BREAST-FEEDING: This drug is found in breast milk. The potential effects of exposure to this drug on a breast-feeding infant are not known. Nursing mothers taking this drug should use caution when breast-feeding due to the potential sedative effects of the drug.

BRAND NAME: **Fiorinal**
GENERIC NAME: **Combination product containing aspirin, butalbital, and caffeine**
USES: **To treat tension headache and for pain relief**
FDA PREGNANCY CATEGORY: **C**

VIRTUALLY NO RISK	SLIGHT RISK	MODERATE RISK	STRONG RISK	EXTREME RISK

Fiorinal is a combination of three ingredients—butalbital, aspirin, and caffeine. When used in small amounts, caffeine has not been associated with fetal malformations or miscarriages. High doses of caffeine may be responsible for miscarriage, difficulty in becoming pregnant, and infertility. Increased heart rate and breathing rate have been observed in a fetus who has been exposed to high amounts of caffeine. Butalbital is a barbiturate drug usually used to treat pain. No adequate studies have been conducted in animals to determine if butalbital causes birth defects. In one human study, a small percentage of birth defects, including cardiovascular problems and spina bifida, was reported. In 112 newborns exposed to butalbital during the first trimester, there were no malformations reported. Butalbital should not be considered for long-term use or in high doses near the end of pregnancy because of its potential to cause withdrawal symptoms in newborns. Aspirin is potentially the most common and most dangerous drug taken during pregnancy. In general, long-term use should be avoided because it can cause an increase in the risk of bleeding in the fetus at any time. High doses (650mg to 1,000mg) should be avoided, especially during the last trimester of pregnancy. Lower doses should also be avoided in the last trimester because they have been associated with heart problems in the fetus. Therefore, this combination product should not be taken during pregnancy, and especially not during the last three months of pregnancy.

BREAST-FEEDING: This drug is found in breast milk and may be harmful to a breast-feeding infant. This drug should not be taken by nursing mothers.

BRAND NAME: **Flagyl**
GENERIC NAME: **metronidazole**
USES: **To treat protozoal infections, bacterial infections, and trichomoniasis**
FDA PREGNANCY CATEGORY: **B**

VIRTUALLY NO RISK	SLIGHT RISK	MODERATE RISK	STRONG RISK	EXTREME RISK

The use of this drug during pregnancy is very controversial. Several studies and case reports have described the safe use of this drug during pregnancy. However, some reports indicate that an increased chance of birth defects in the fetus may occur when the drug is used during the first trimester of pregnancy. As of May 1987, the Food and Drug Administration had received reports of 27 adverse effects to the fetus when used during pregnancy. These included miscarriages, limb defects, and brain defects. The FDA cannot be completely sure that this drug and not some other factor directly caused these defects. However, the presence of these defects warrants some caution when using the drug during pregnancy. In summary, the use of this drug during pregnancy is controversial and caution should be used. The risks of using the drug should be weighed against the potential harm to the fetus. The Centers for Disease Control suggest that the drug should not be used during the first trimester of pregnancy. A large single dose of Flagyl, a common dosing regimen, should definitely be avoided. Smaller, more frequent doses should be used instead, when necessary.

BREAST-FEEDING: This drug is found in breast milk and may be harmful to a breast-feeding infant. The American Academy of Pediatrics recommends that breast-feeding should be discontinued until 24 to 48 hours after the mother takes the last dose of drug.

BRAND NAME: **Flexeril**
GENERIC NAME: **cyclobenzaprine**
USES: **To treat muscle spasms**
FDA PREGNANCY CATEGORY: **B**

VIRTUALLY NO RISK	SLIGHT RISK	MODERATE RISK	STRONG RISK	EXTREME RISK
▒	▒			

Used as a muscle relaxant, this drug has not been shown to cause birth defects in mice, rats, or rabbits. With no published information on the use of this agent during pregnancy in humans, caution should be used when taking this medication.

BREAST-FEEDING: It is not known whether the drug is found in breast milk. Caution should be used when breast-feeding.

BRAND NAME: **Flonase**

GENERIC NAME: **fluticasone**

USES: **To treat nasal allergies**

FDA PREGNANCY CATEGORY: **C**

VIRTUALLY NO RISK	SLIGHT RISK	MODERATE RISK	STRONG RISK	EXTREME RISK

Flonase is a corticosteroid inhaled through the nose for the treatment of allergies and runny nose. There are no studies in humans concerning the use of Flonase in pregnancy. Studies in rats and mice given shots of fluticasone showed delayed growth of the fetus, cleft palate, and improper skull growth. Fluticasone has been shown to cross the placenta in rats and rabbits, and should not be used in pregnancy unless its benefits outweigh its risks to the fetus.

BREAST-FEEDING: It is not known whether the drug is found in breast milk. Caution should be used when breast-feeding.

BRAND NAME: **Flovent**

GENERIC NAME: **fluticasone**

See entry for **Flonase**

BRAND NAME: **Floxin**

GENERIC NAME: **ofloxacin**

USES: **To treat bacterial infections**

FDA PREGNANCY CATEGORY: **C**

VIRTUALLY NO RISK	SLIGHT RISK	MODERATE RISK	STRONG RISK	EXTREME RISK

Floxin is an anti-infective that is generally not recommended for use during pregnancy. Several studies of pregnant women taking Floxin have shown birth defects, including water on the brain, hernias, and heart malformations in the fetus. Studies have also shown damage to the cartilage in various joints in immature rats and dogs, and some joint abnormalities have been noted in children exposed to this category of antibacterial during pregnancy. Although these results do not establish a definite relationship between drug exposure and birth defects, Floxin should absolutely not be taken during the first trimester because of the abnormalities observed in animals when exposed to this type of drug during this time. To be on the safe side, Floxin should be avoided throughout the rest of pregnancy as well.

BREAST-FEEDING: This drug is found in breast milk and may be harmful to a breast-feeding infant. This drug should not be taken by nursing mothers.

BRAND NAME: **Gabitril**
GENERIC NAME: **tiagabine**
USES: **To manage seizures**
FDA PREGNANCY CATEGORY: **C**

VIRTUALLY NO RISK	SLIGHT RISK	MODERATE RISK	STRONG RISK	EXTREME RISK

Gabitril is a drug used to control seizures in patients with epilepsy. It has been shown to cause birth defects in both rats and rabbits. In rats given a dose almost 16 times greater than the normal human dose, defects in the skull, face, and skeleton were observed in the offspring. There are no studies of pregnant women that examine the relationship between Gabitril and birth defects. Gabitril is not recommended for use in pregnancy.

BREAST-FEEDING: It is not known whether the drug is found in breast milk. Extreme caution should be used when breast-feeding due to the potential to cause serious adverse effects in the infant.

BRAND NAME: **Glucophage**

GENERIC NAME: **metformin**

USES: **To treat diabetes**

FDA PREGNANCY CATEGORY: **B**

VIRTUALLY NO RISK	SLIGHT RISK	MODERATE RISK	STRONG RISK	EXTREME RISK

Glucophage is an oral drug used to treat high blood sugar in diabetic patients. In general, this medication should not be a first-line treatment for diabetes during pregnancy. In some studies, birth defects have been reported with the use of Glucophage alone and include malformations of the heart, and a missing bone in the spine. In combination with other oral medications to control blood sugar, such as glyburide, the risk for birth defects seems to increase. Jaundice and the need for blood transfusions was also seen in infants exposed to these drugs during pregnancy. Glucophage should not be used to control blood sugar in diabetic patients who are pregnant. Insulin would be the drug of choice for such patients during pregnancy.

BREAST-FEEDING: It is not known whether the drug is found in breast milk. Caution should be used when breast-feeding.

BRAND NAME: **Glucotrol XL**

GENERIC NAME: **glipizide**

USES: **To treat diabetes**

FDA PREGNANCY CATEGORY: **C**

VIRTUALLY NO RISK	SLIGHT RISK	MODERATE RISK	STRONG RISK	EXTREME RISK

Glucotrol XL is an oral drug used to control the blood sugar of diabetic patients. Glucotrol XL is not the drug of choice for such pregnant patients. In studies conducted in pregnant mothers who received oral medications—including Glucotrol XL—to control their blood sugar, a large percentage of the infants showed one or more malformations. These malformations included deformities of the face, heart, and central nervous system. Although a high percentage of birth defects resulted from the mothers who took the drugs, researchers also believe that poor control of the mother's blood sugar could also have contributed to these birth defects. Glucotrol XL should not be used by diabetic patients who are pregnant; instead insulin should be used to control blood sugar levels.

BREAST-FEEDING: It is not known whether the drug is found in breast milk. Caution should be used when breast-feeding.

BRAND NAME: **Glynase**
GENERIC NAME: **glyburide (micronized)**
See entry for **DiaBeta**

BRAND NAME: **Habitrol**
GENERIC NAME: **nicotine transdermal patch**
USES: **An aid to help quit smoking**
FDA PREGNANCY CATEGORY: **D**

VIRTUALLY NO RISK	SLIGHT RISK	MODERATE RISK	STRONG RISK	EXTREME RISK

Nicotine is harmful to the fetus. Animal and human studies have shown many adverse effects, including preterm births, decreased birth weight, increased heart rate, and increased risk of abortion and stillbirth. When nicotine is used during the third trimester, breathing problems may be noted in the fetus. This drug is transferred via the placenta, and the fetus is exposed to higher amounts of it than the pregnant mother. Even though this drug is harmful to the fetus, in some cases it may helpful. When a heavy smoker is trying to quit, using the transdermal patch may outweigh the risks of continued smoking during pregnancy. Each individual should be evaluated to see if the patch is more beneficial than heavy smoking.

BREAST-FEEDING: This drug is found in breast milk. The potential effects of exposure to this drug on a breast-feeding infant are not known. Women taking this drug should use caution when breast-feeding.

BRAND NAME: **Haldol**

GENERIC NAME: **haloperidol**

USES: **To help control psychotic disorders and severe behavioral problems**

FDA PREGNANCY CATEGORY: **C**

VIRTUALLY NO RISK	SLIGHT RISK	MODERATE RISK	STRONG RISK	EXTREME RISK

Isolated cases of birth defects have been reported, but no definite connection to this drug has been established. Some risks have been associated with the use of high doses of this drug during pregnancy. Cases of arm and leg defects have been observed in first-trimester exposure, which may warrant additional caution. This drug has been used during labor without any effects on the newborn. It is suggested that the use of this drug should be limited to psychotic patients needing long-term therapy. As long as this drug is used correctly, the benefit to the mother may outweigh the risk to the fetus.

BREAST-FEEDING: This drug is found in breast milk and may be harmful to a breast-feeding infant. This drug should not be taken by nursing mothers.

BRAND NAME: **Humibid LA**

GENERIC NAME: **guaifenesin**

USES: **To relieve chest congestion**

FDA PREGNANCY CATEGORY: **C**

VIRTUALLY NO RISK	SLIGHT RISK	MODERATE RISK	STRONG RISK	EXTREME RISK

No animal studies are available and one human pregnancy study has been performed using this drug. The data did not show a definite relationship between birth defects and guaifenesin. This agent may be fairly safe and is probably the preferred expectorant in pregnant asthmatic patients. The medical community considers its effectiveness as an expectorant questionable. Drinking lots of water is the preferred expectorant for pregnant women.

BREAST-FEEDING: It is not known whether the drug is found in breast milk. Caution should be used when breast-feeding.

BRAND NAME: **Humulin N**

GENERIC NAME: **insulin**

USES: **To treat diabetes**

FDA PREGNANCY CATEGORY: **B**

VIRTUALLY NO RISK	SLIGHT RISK	MODERATE RISK	STRONG RISK	EXTREME RISK

Insulin is the drug of choice in treating diabetes during pregnancy. Insulin is usually taken through a subcutaneous injection (a shot given into the fatty tissue). Although some other drugs are available in tablet formulations to help control blood sugar, their risk for causing birth defects is much higher. Insulin is a naturally occurring hormone that is produced in the pancreas. Infants born to diabetic mothers are at a 3 to 5 times higher risk for malformations and birth defects than infants born to nondiabetic mothers. These high rates of birth defects seem to be related to poor blood sugar control, especially in the first trimester of pregnancy. Insulin should be used by pregnant women who are diabetic or who have increased blood sugar levels.

BREAST-FEEDING: This drug is not found in breast milk. Women may safely breast-feed while taking this drug.

BRAND NAME: **Hytrin**
GENERIC NAME: **terazosin**
USES: **To treat high blood pressure**
FDA PREGNANCY CATEGORY: **C**

VIRTUALLY NO RISK	SLIGHT RISK	MODERATE RISK	STRONG RISK	EXTREME RISK

Hytrin is a drug used to treat high blood pressure. When studied in rats and rabbits at doses much higher than the maximum recommended human dose, no developmental abnormalities were seen. No reports studying the effects of Hytrin in pregnant women exist. This drug should only be used in pregnancy if its benefits strongly outweigh its potential risks to the fetus.

BREAST-FEEDING: It is not known whether the drug is found in breast milk. Extreme caution should be used when breast-feeding.

BRAND NAME: **Hyzaar**
GENERIC NAME: **Combination product containing losartan and hydrochlorothiazide**
USES: **To treat high blood pressure and alleviate fluid retention due to congestive heart failure, kidney disease, or cirrhosis of the liver**
FDA PREGNANCY CATEGORY: **D**

VIRTUALLY NO RISK	SLIGHT RISK	MODERATE RISK	STRONG RISK	EXTREME RISK

The losartan component of this combination product is assumed to cause birth defects because of its close relationship to such drugs as Vasotec and Capoten. Birth defects have been reported when used in the second and third trimesters. Some of the effects include low blood pressure, renal problems, anemia, and low red blood cell counts. Limb and facial deformities are also a possibility, along with lung development problems. A possibility exists for stunted growth and premature birth. Exposure during the first trimester may be safer. The hydrochlorothiazide component has also been associated with fetal problems. Some of these include decreased birth weight, water depletion, decreased blood sugar, jaundice, and possibly death. With the risks associated with this drug, other treatment options should be used first. This drug should be used as a last resort in treating high blood pressure.

BREAST-FEEDING: This drug is found in breast milk. The potential effects of exposure to this drug on a breast-feeding infant are not known. Nursing mothers taking this drug should use caution when breast-feeding.

BRAND NAME: **Imitrex**
GENERIC NAME: **sumatriptan**
USES: **To treat migraines**
FDA PREGNANCY CATEGORY: **C**

VIRTUALLY NO RISK	SLIGHT RISK	MODERATE RISK	STRONG RISK	EXTREME RISK

The number of birth defects reported with first-trimester exposure to this drug appears to be unclear. A common cause cannot be identified because there is not a consistent pattern among the defects. Some of the defects include abnormal head size, cleft palate, hernia, and abnormal development. The safety of this product is hard to assess, so it is suggested that if this product is to be used, extreme caution should be taken due to potential cardiovascular effects. The benefits must clearly outweigh the risks involved.

BREAST-FEEDING: This drug is found in breast milk. The potential effects of exposure to this drug on a breast-feeding infant are not known. Nursing mothers taking this drug should use extreme caution when breast-feeding.

BRAND NAME: **Inderal**
GENERIC NAME: **propranolol**
USES: **To treat high blood pressure, irregular heartbeat, angina; for use after heart attacks; and to prevent migraine**
FDA PREGNANCY CATEGORY: **C**

VIRTUALLY NO RISK	SLIGHT RISK	MODERATE RISK	STRONG RISK	EXTREME RISK

This drug is part of the family known as the beta-blockers. It can be used for fetal and maternal problems throughout pregnancy. The drug is not a teratogen, but toxicity is a concern. Some of the beta-blockers, including Inderal, are known to cause stunted growth and decreased birth weight. When the drug is given during the second trimester, the greatest reduction in birth weight occurs. Even though growth retardation is a concern, the benefits for the pregnant mother may outweigh the risks to the fetus. This must be examined on an individual basis. If this agent is used in the second or third trimesters, the risk to the fetus may increase.

BREAST-FEEDING: This drug is found in breast milk. The potential effects of exposure to this drug on a breast-feeding infant are not known. Nursing mothers taking this drug should use caution when breast-feeding.

BRAND NAME: **Intal**

GENERIC NAME: **cromolyn sodium**

USES: **To prevent asthma attacks and bronchospasms**

FDA PREGNANCY CATEGORY: **B**

VIRTUALLY NO RISK	SLIGHT RISK	MODERATE RISK	STRONG RISK	EXTREME RISK
▓	▓			

Intal is used to prevent asthma attacks and is usually considered safe for use in pregnant women. Although some studies have been conducted in mothers who received cromolyn sodium and had children with birth defects, the percentage was very small and could not be linked directly to the drug. The birth defects could have been caused by other drugs, disease states, or the genetics of the parents.

BREAST-FEEDING: It is not known whether the drug is found in breast milk. Some caution should be used when breast-feeding.

BRAND NAME: **K-Dur**

GENERIC NAME: **potassium (as chloride)**

USES: **To treat low potassium levels**

FDA PREGNANCY CATEGORY: **C**

VIRTUALLY NO RISK	SLIGHT RISK	MODERATE RISK	STRONG RISK	EXTREME RISK
▓	▓	▓		

Potassium is normally found in the body. Some people, including pregnant women, may have decreased levels and need to replace it. It is important to know that high or low blood levels of potassium can harm the mother and the fetus. Therefore, the potassium blood levels of the mother should be monitored closely in order to prevent any birth defects. K-Dur should be used with caution and only under the direction of a physician during pregnancy.

BREAST-FEEDING: This drug is found in breast milk. The American Academy of Pediatrics considers this drug to be compatible with breast-feeding. As with all drugs, some caution should still be exercised.

BRAND NAME: **Keflex**

GENERIC NAME: **cephalexin**

USES: **To treat bacterial infections**

FDA PREGNANCY CATEGORY: **B**

VIRTUALLY NO RISK	SLIGHT RISK	MODERATE RISK	STRONG RISK	EXTREME RISK

Keflex is an oral antibiotic that is generally considered safe for use during pregnancy. Several studies have been published that showed no birth defects in the infants. However, as with any drug, Keflex should be used with some caution during pregnancy.

BREAST-FEEDING: This drug is found in breast milk. The potential effects of exposure to this drug on a breast-feeding infant are not known. However, the drug should be considered fairly safe to use during breast-feeding.

BRAND NAME: **Klonopin**

GENERIC NAME: **clonazepam**

USES: **To treat epilepsy and seizures**

FDA PREGNANCY CATEGORY: **D**

VIRTUALLY NO RISK	SLIGHT RISK	MODERATE RISK	STRONG RISK	EXTREME RISK

Toxicity has been reported with the use of Klonopin during pregnancy. Some of these problems include a lack of oxygen to the newborn resulting in a bluish-colored baby, a lack of spontaneous breathing, a minimal response from the baby, and tiredness. Problems with breathing have been shown in newborns up until ten weeks of age. Lethargy or tiredness has been seen in newborns for up to five days. Fetal exposure to this drug may cause addiction, so close monitoring is needed. The baby may suffer from withdrawal effects upon delivery, which include shakiness, diarrhea, vomiting, and irritability. This drug does cross the placenta and can cause "floppy infant syndrome." Floppy infant syndrome occurs at birth and its symptoms include tiredness and sucking difficulties. With minimal information available, this drug should be avoided during pregnancy due to its potential adverse effects on the fetus.

BREAST-FEEDING: This drug is found in breast milk and may be harmful to a breast-feeding infant. This drug should not be taken by nursing mothers.

BRAND NAME: **Lamictal**
GENERIC NAME: **lamotrigine**
USES: **To treat epilepsy and prevent seizures**
FDA PREGNANCY CATEGORY: **C**

VIRTUALLY NO RISK	SLIGHT RISK	MODERATE RISK	STRONG RISK	EXTREME RISK

Lamictal is a drug used to prevent seizures in epileptic patients. In numerous case studies, birth defects have been reported and include miscarriage, various malformations—including extra bones and deformities in the heart—and various problems in the brain. Conditions other than birth defects were noticed in newborns, and included jaundice, increased rate of breathing, and delayed growth. Due to the very serious birth defects that could be caused by this drug, it is not recommended for use in pregnancy unless its benefits strongly outweigh its potential risks to the fetus.

BREAST-FEEDING: This drug is found in breast milk. The potential effects of exposure to this drug on a breast-feeding infant are not known. Nursing mothers taking this drug should use extreme caution when breast-feeding.

BRAND NAME: **Lamisil**

GENERIC NAME: **terbinafine**

USES: **To treat fungal infections (mainly ringworm, jock itch in men, athlete's foot, toenail and fingernail fungus)**

FDA PREGNANCY CATEGORY: **B**

VIRTUALLY NO RISK	SLIGHT RISK	MODERATE RISK	STRONG RISK	EXTREME RISK

Lamisil is an oral and topical drug used to treat toenail and fingernail fungus and athlete's foot. In studies conducted in rats and rabbits given doses up to 9 and 12 times the maximum recommended human daily dose, no adverse effects on the fetus were observed. No studies have been done in humans to look at the effects of using or taking Lamisil during pregnancy. Lamisil should be used with some caution during pregnancy.

BREAST-FEEDING: This drug is found in breast milk. The manufacturer recommends that this drug should not be taken while breast-feeding.

BRAND NAME: **Lanoxin**

GENERIC NAME: **digoxin**

USES: **To treat congestive heart failure, irregular heartbeat, and fast heartbeat**

FDA PREGNANCY CATEGORY: **C**

VIRTUALLY NO RISK	SLIGHT RISK	MODERATE RISK	STRONG RISK	EXTREME RISK

Currently no cases of birth defects have been found when Lanoxin is used as indicated during pregnancy. This drug can be used for heart problems in the mother or the fetus. When taken appropriately and the pregnant woman is regularly monitored, this drug is fairly safe. However, in an overdose, fetal toxicity can occur and result in death. When taking this drug during pregnancy, caution and careful monitoring should be used to minimize harmful effects to the baby.

BREAST-FEEDING: This drug is found in breast milk. The potential effects of exposure to this drug on a breast-feeding infant are not known. Nursing mothers taking this drug should use caution when breast-feeding.

BRAND NAME: **Lasix**
GENERIC NAME: **furosemide**
Similar to **Bumex;** see entry for **Bumex**

BRAND NAME: **Lescol**
GENERIC NAME: **fluvastatin**
Similar to **Mevacor;** see entry for **Mevacor**

BRAND NAME: **Levaquin**
GENERIC NAME: **levofloxacin**
Similar to **Floxin;** see entry for **Floxin**

BRAND NAME: **Levoxyl**
GENERIC NAME: **levothyroxine**
USES: **Thyroid hormone replacement therapy**
FDA PREGNANCY CATEGORY: **A**

VIRTUALLY NO RISK	SLIGHT RISK	MODERATE RISK	STRONG RISK	EXTREME RISK

Levoxyl is a natural thyroid hormone that is produced by both the mother and the fetus. Most research claims that very little of the drug crosses the placenta. In a large study looking at infants exposed to thyroid hormone during the first trimester, some cardiovascular problems and Down syndrome were reported. There were not enough cases to directly link these birth defects to the thyroid hormone. Mothers who do not have enough thyroid hormone have also been shown to have poor pregnancy outcomes. Although data is not complete, the use of thyroid hormone during pregnancy is safe when properly monitored.

BREAST-FEEDING: This drug is found in breast milk. The potential effects of exposure to this drug on a breast-feeding infant are not known. Nursing mothers taking this drug should use caution when breast-feeding.

BRAND NAME: **Levsin**
GENERIC NAME: **hyoscyamine**
USES: **To treat peptic ulcers, stomach spasms, and irritable bowel syndrome**
FDA PREGNANCY CATEGORY: **C**

VIRTUALLY NO RISK	SLIGHT RISK	MODERATE RISK	STRONG RISK	EXTREME RISK

There are no published reports on the use of Levsin during pregnancy. In a large observational study, a small percentage of infants exposed to Levsin in the first trimester had major birth defects, with the most common being multiple fingers/toes and decreased number of limbs. The use of Levsin in pregnancy is not recommended because of a lack of safety data in human subjects.

BREAST-FEEDING: This drug is found in breast milk. The potential effects of exposure to this drug on a breast-feeding infant are not known. Nursing mothers taking this drug should use caution when breast-feeding.

BRAND NAME: **Lipitor**

GENERIC NAME: **atorvastatin**

USES: **To treat high cholesterol**

FDA PREGNANCY CATEGORY: **X**

VIRTUALLY NO RISK	SLIGHT RISK	MODERATE RISK	STRONG RISK	EXTREME RISK

In rats and rabbits given large doses, no birth defects or adverse effects were reported with the use of this drug. When other drugs in this class, such as Mevacor (lovastatin), were administered to pregnant women, birth defects and adverse effects were reported. These defects included cleft lip, outgrowths from the hand, and clubfoot. Also, some adverse effects reported include miscarriage, breathing problems, infection, and heart problems. Because this drug has no effect on the short-term treatment of lowering cholesterol and because of the adverse effects and birth defects reported, this drug should not be used during pregnancy due to the possibility of harm to the fetus.

BREAST-FEEDING: This drug is found in breast milk and may be harmful to a breast-feeding infant. This drug should not be taken by nursing mothers.

BRAND NAME: **Lithobid**

GENERIC NAME: **lithium carbonate**

USES: **To treat bipolar disorder and manic episodes**

FDA PREGNANCY CATEGORY: **D**

VIRTUALLY NO RISK	SLIGHT RISK	MODERATE RISK	STRONG RISK	EXTREME RISK

Lithobid is used to treat various manic and manic-depressive disorders. Lithobid freely crosses the placenta and has been associated with an increased number of birth defects, especially of the cardiovascular system. Some of these cardiovascular defects include problems with the chambers and valves of the heart. Other potential adverse effects to the fetus include slow heart rate, increased liver size, bleeding in the stomach and intestine, seizures, and shock. Lithobid should not be used during pregnancy unless its benefits significantly outweigh the serious risk of adverse effects to the fetus.

BREAST-FEEDING: This drug is found in breast milk and may be harmful to a breast-feeding infant. Lithobid should not be taken by nursing mothers.

BRAND NAME: **Lodine**

GENERIC NAME: **etodolac**

USES: **For treatment of arthritis and for pain relief**

FDA PREGNANCY CATEGORY: **C**

VIRTUALLY NO RISK	SLIGHT RISK	MODERATE RISK	STRONG RISK	EXTREME RISK

Lodine is a nonsteroidal anti-inflammatory drug (NSAID) used to treat generalized pain. No reports concerning the use of Lodine in humans are available. Lodine use in rats has been shown to increase the chances of labor problems, make the pregnancy longer, and decrease survival in the pups. Women who are trying to conceive should not take Lodine because it may block the implantation of the fertilized egg. Lodine should not be given in the third trimester or near delivery because it may inhibit the natural labor process, cause high blood pressure in the lungs of the fetus, or decrease kidney function in the fetus.

BREAST-FEEDING: This drug is found in breast milk. The potential effects of exposure to this drug on a breast-feeding infant are not known. Nursing mothers taking this drug should use caution when breast-feeding.

BRAND NAME: **Loestrin Fe 1.5/30**

GENERIC NAME: **Combination product containing norethindrone and ethinyl estradiol**

Similar to **Alesse-28;** see entry for **Alesse-28**

BRAND NAME: **Lomotil**

GENERIC NAME: **Combination product containing diphenoxylate and atropine**

USES: **To treat diarrhea**

FDA PREGNANCY CATEGORY: **C**

VIRTUALLY NO RISK	SLIGHT RISK	MODERATE RISK	STRONG RISK	EXTREME RISK
▓▓▓▓▓▓	▓▓▓▓▓▓	▓▓▓▓▓▓		

Lomotil is a combination of two products used to treat diarrhea—diphenoxylate and atropine. Diphenoxylate is a narcotic pain reliever used only in combination products to discourage overdosage. In one study, no adverse effects were seen after first-trimester exposure to diphenoxylate. In a larger observational study, a small percentage of birth defects, including cardiovascular defects and spina bifida, were seen. The small percentage of birth defects does not prove that these were caused by the use of diphenoxylate. Atropine easily crosses the placenta and has been shown to decrease fetal breathing. In a Michigan study, a small percentage of birth defects was present in infants who had been exposed to atropine during the first trimester. The most common defect was a decrease in the number of arms/legs. Other factors, including diseases of the mother and other drug use, could also have caused these birth defects. This combination product is not recommended for use in pregnancy unless its benefits strongly outweigh its risks to the fetus.

BREAST-FEEDING: This drug is found in breast milk and may be harmful to a breast-feeding infant. This drug should not be taken by nursing mothers.

BRAND NAME: **Lo/Orral**

GENERIC NAME: **Combination product containing norgestrel and ethinyl estradiol**

Similar to **Alesse-28;** see entry for **Alesse-28**

BRAND NAME: **Lopressor**

GENERIC NAME: **metoprolol tartrate**

USES: **To treat high blood pressure and angina, and for use after a heart attack to reduce the risk of recurrent heart attack**

FDA PREGNANCY CATEGORY: **C**

VIRTUALLY NO RISK	SLIGHT RISK	MODERATE RISK	STRONG RISK	EXTREME RISK

This drug belongs to the family known as beta-blockers. It can be used for serious fetal and maternal problems throughout pregnancy. The drug is not known to cause birth defects, but information is limited. Some of the beta-blockers are believed to cause stunted growth and decreased heart rate. Other beta-blockers have shown a decrease in fetal and placental weight. When the drug is taken in the second trimester, the greatest reduction in birth weight occurs. Even though growth retardation is a concern, the benefits for the pregnant mother may outweigh the risks to the fetus, which must be examined on an individual basis. If this agent is used in the second or third trimesters, an increased risk to the fetus may occur. The long-term effects of the use of beta-blockers, including Lopressor, have not been studied. If its use is warranted during pregnancy, caution should be taken.

BREAST-FEEDING: This drug is found in breast milk. The potential effects of exposure to this drug on a breast-feeding infant are not known. Nursing mothers taking this drug should use caution when breast-feeding.

BRAND NAME: **Lorabid**

GENERIC NAME: **loracarbef**

USES: **To treat bacterial infections**

FDA PREGNANCY CATEGORY: **B**

VIRTUALLY NO RISK	SLIGHT RISK	MODERATE RISK	STRONG RISK	EXTREME RISK

Lorabid is an oral antibiotic that is generally considered safe for use in pregnancy. Doses in mice and rabbits of up to 4 times the maximum recommended human dose showed no harm to the fetus or in fertility. No reports concerning the use of Lorabid in human pregnancy are available.

BREAST-FEEDING: It is not known whether the drug is found in breast milk. Some caution should be used when breast-feeding.

BRAND NAME: **Lortab**

GENERIC NAME: **Combination product containing acetaminophen and hydrocodone**

USES: **For relief of moderate to severe pain**

FDA PREGNANCY CATEGORY: **C**

VIRTUALLY NO RISK	SLIGHT RISK	MODERATE RISK	STRONG RISK	EXTREME RISK

The acetaminophen component of this drug is safe during all stages of pregnancy. It is apparently safest for short-term use, because long-term use can cause problems in the infant, such as anemia or a low red blood cell count. However, because of the hydrocodone component, some caution is needed. Some birth defects have been reported with this drug in hamsters. In humans, one study reported malformations when the fetus was exposed during the first trimester, but no concrete evidence was reported. The hydrocodone component of this drug may cause withdrawal in infants if mothers use high doses. If used for prolonged periods or in high doses, risk to the fetus may increase. This drug should be used with extreme caution if taken for long periods of time during pregnancy.

BREAST-FEEDING: This drug is found in breast milk. The potential effects of exposure to this drug on a breast-feeding infant are not known. Nursing mothers taking this drug should use caution when breast-feeding.

BRAND NAME: **Lotensin**
GENERIC NAME: **benazepril**
Similar to **Accupril;** see entry for **Accupril**

BRAND NAME: **Lotrel**
GENERIC NAME: **Combination product containing amlodipine and benazepril**
USES: **To treat high blood pressure**
FDA PREGNANCY CATEGORY: **D**

VIRTUALLY NO RISK	SLIGHT RISK	MODERATE RISK	STRONG RISK	EXTREME RISK

There are no clinical studies regarding the use of this drug during pregnancy. Other agents in this class have caused a malformed fetus, stunted growth, breathing problems, renal problems, and low blood pressure. It is unclear whether exposure to agents in this class during the first trimester causes birth defects. They may cause birth defects when used during the second or third trimester of pregnancy. Lotrel should be used with extreme caution during pregnancy.

BREAST-FEEDING: It is not known whether the drug is found in breast milk. Caution should be used when breast-feeding.

BRAND NAME: **Lotrisone**

GENERIC NAME: **Combination product containing clotrimazole and betamethasone dipropionate**

USES: **To treat fungal infections (mainly ringworm, jock itch in men, and athlete's foot)**

FDA PREGNANCY CATEGORY: **C**

VIRTUALLY NO RISK	SLIGHT RISK	MODERATE RISK	STRONG RISK	EXTREME RISK

This topical combination product has no reports of birth defects associated with its use. The clotrimazole component has no adverse effects associated with its use. The betamethasone component usually shows more of a benefit to the mother than a risk to the fetus when used in humans during pregnancy. Low birth weight is a possibility, but no birth defects have been reported. However, due to the lack of clinical studies, this drug should be used with some caution.

BREAST-FEEDING: It is not known whether the drug is found in breast milk. Some caution should be used when breast-feeding.

BRAND NAME: **Lozol**

GENERIC NAME: **indapamide**

USES: **To treat fluid retention due to congestive heart failure, kidney disease, or cirrhosis of the liver and to treat high blood pressure**

FDA PREGNANCY CATEGORY: **B**

VIRTUALLY NO RISK	SLIGHT RISK	MODERATE RISK	STRONG RISK	EXTREME RISK

There is little information available regarding the use of Lozol during pregnancy. In rats and rabbits taking high doses, birth defects were not found, except for stunted growth. Therefore, this drug may be safe to use during pregnancy, but more information is needed and some caution should be used.

BREAST-FEEDING: It is not known whether the drug is found in breast milk. Caution should be used when breast-feeding.

BRAND NAME: **Luvox**

GENERIC NAME: **fluvoxamine**

USES: **To treat obsessive-compulsive disorder and depression**

FDA PREGNANCY CATEGORY: **C**

VIRTUALLY NO RISK	SLIGHT RISK	MODERATE RISK	STRONG RISK	EXTREME RISK

Luvox is a drug used to treat depression and obsessive-compulsive disorder. When rats were dosed at 2 to 4 times the maximum recommended human dose, decreased birth weight and increased stillbirth occurred. No records are currently available concerning the use of Luvox in humans. Long-term studies are needed to determine its effects. Luvox is not recommended for use in pregnancy unless its benefits strongly outweigh the risks to the fetus.

BREAST-FEEDING: This drug is found in breast milk. The potential effects of exposure to this drug on a breast-feeding infant are not known. Nursing mothers taking this drug should use caution when breast-feeding.

BRAND NAME: **Macrobid**

GENERIC NAME: **nitrofurantoin**

USES: **To treat urinary tract infections**

FDA PREGNANCY CATEGORY: **B**

VIRTUALLY NO RISK	SLIGHT RISK	MODERATE RISK	STRONG RISK	EXTREME RISK

The use of Macrobid in rats and rabbits has produced no adverse effects in their fetuses. In one published study of humans, 91 patients receiving Macrobid during pregnancy showed no adverse effects in any of the infants. Macrobid has been shown to cause anemia (decrease in red blood cells) in patients who are deficient in a certain enzyme, and this enzyme is also low in newborn children. Therefore, it is recommended to avoid the use of Macrobid near the time of delivery, and it should be used with some caution at other times during pregnancy.

BREAST-FEEDING: This drug is found in breast milk. The American Academy of Pediatrics considers this drug to be compatible with breast-feeding. As with all drugs, some caution should still be used.

BRAND NAME: **Macrodantin**
GENERIC NAME: **nitrofurantoin**
See entry for **Macrobid**

BRAND NAME: **Maxzide**
GENERIC NAME: **Combination product containing triamterene and hydrochlorothiazide**
See entry for **Dyazide**

BRAND NAME: **Meridia**
GENERIC NAME: **sibutramine**
USES: **For weight loss**
FDA PREGNANCY CATEGORY: **C**

VIRTUALLY NO RISK	SLIGHT RISK	MODERATE RISK	STRONG RISK	EXTREME RISK

When Meridia was studied in rats, no evidence of birth defects was found. However, when this drug was given to pregnant rabbits at 5 times the human dose, toxicities occurred including heart problems. Adequate studies are not available regarding the use of this drug during pregnancy in humans. Women who are pregnant should never try to lose weight with prescription drugs. Meridia should be avoided during pregnancy.

BREAST-FEEDING: This drug is found in breast milk and may be harmful to a breast-feeding infant. This drug should not be taken by nursing mothers.

BRAND NAME: **MetroGel Vaginal**
GENERIC NAME: **metronidazole**
USES: **To treat bacterial vaginal infections**
FDA PREGNANCY CATEGORY: **B**

VIRTUALLY NO RISK	SLIGHT RISK	MODERATE RISK	STRONG RISK	EXTREME RISK

The use of MetroGel in pregnancy is a topic of debate. The drug has been shown to cause mutations in bacteria and to be a cancer-causing agent in rodents; however, this has not been proven in humans. Several reports to the FDA have included adverse events, including miscarriage, defects in the fetal brain and arms/legs, and cardiovascular defects. Other studies have not linked the use of MetroGel with birth defects, but the different opinions show a need for caution with MetroGel in pregnancy. MetroGel is not recommended for use during pregnancy, especially during the first trimester. At other times during the pregnancy, the benefits of using MetroGel should strongly outweigh the potential adverse effects to the fetus.

BREAST-FEEDING: This drug is found in breast milk. The potential effects of exposure to this drug on a breast-feeding infant are not known; therefore nursing mothers taking this drug should use extreme caution when breast-feeding.

BRAND NAME: **Mevacor**

GENERIC NAME: **lovastatin**

USES: **To treat high cholesterol**

FDA PREGNANCY CATEGORY: **X**

VIRTUALLY NO RISK	SLIGHT RISK	MODERATE RISK	STRONG RISK	EXTREME RISK

Mevacor has been shown to cause birth defects in rats and mice, including bone malformation and decreased fetal weight. In women taking this drug along with other drugs during pregnancy, heart defects, brain dysfunction, a missing thumb, spinal column defects, and spina bifida have occurred. The cause of these birth defects is unknown, but the potential for it to be related to Mevacor is significant. Also, there is no benefit to the pregnant woman to use this drug during pregnancy. High levels of cholesterol for 9 months should not adversely affect long-term cardiovascular health in most women. Due to the absence of benefit and the possibility of causing birth defects, this drug should never be used during pregnancy.

BREAST-FEEDING: This drug is found in breast milk and may be harmful to a breast-feeding infant. This drug should not be taken by nursing mothers.

BRAND NAME: **Micronase**

GENERIC NAME: **glyburide**

See entry for **DiaBeta**

BRAND NAME: **Minocin**

GENERIC NAME: **minocycline**

USES: **To treat bacterial infections and acne**

FDA PREGNANCY CATEGORY: **D**

VIRTUALLY NO RISK	SLIGHT RISK	MODERATE RISK	STRONG RISK	EXTREME RISK

The use of Minocin during pregnancy is not recommended due to many possible adverse effects to the fetus. Problems associated with the use of Minocin include a discoloration of the teeth, bone development problems, and liver toxicity in the mother. Congenital effects seen with the use of Minocin include cardiovascular defects and oral clefts. Because of the very high potential for causing birth defects in the fetus, this drug should not be used during pregnancy.

BREAST-FEEDING: This drug is found in breast milk. The American Academy of Pediatrics considers this drug to be compatible with breast-feeding. As with all drugs, some caution should still be used.

BRAND NAME: **Monopril**
GENERIC NAME: **fosinopril**
Similar to **Accupril;** see entry for **Accupril**

BRAND NAME: **Motrin**
GENERIC NAME: **ibuprofen**
USES: **To treat arthritis; for pain relief, fever, and menstrual pain**
FDA PREGNANCY CATEGORY: **B**

VIRTUALLY NO RISK	SLIGHT RISK	MODERATE RISK	STRONG RISK	EXTREME RISK

No well-documented cases have been found that link Motrin to birth defects. Some defects have been reported, such as cerebral palsy and a rotated palate. However, these mothers were also on other medications and these effects cannot be solely linked to Motrin. It should be avoided by those trying to conceive because this drug can block implantation. When used near delivery or in the third trimester, Motrin is classified as a very risky drug because of the possible increase in blood pressure in the infant's lungs. This agent has also been shown to prolong pregnancies and slow down labor. Motrin should be used with caution during pregnancy, as safer options exist for pain and fever reduction.

BREAST-FEEDING: This drug is found in breast milk. The American Academy of Pediatrics considers this drug to be compatible with breast-feeding. As with all drugs, some caution should still be used.

BRAND NAME: **Naprosyn**
GENERIC NAME: **naproxen**
USES: **Arthritis, pain relief, and menstrual pain**
FDA PREGNANCY CATEGORY: **B**

VIRTUALLY NO RISK	SLIGHT RISK	MODERATE RISK	STRONG RISK	EXTREME RISK

Some defects have been reported, such as cerebral palsy and a rotated palate. However, these mothers were also on other medications and these effects cannot be solely linked to Naprosyn. It should be avoided by those trying to conceive because Naprosyn can block egg implantation. When used near delivery or in the third trimester, it is classified as a very risky drug because of the possible increase in blood pressure in the infant's lungs. This agent has also been shown to prolong pregnancies and slow down labor. Naprosyn should be used with caution during pregnancy, as safer options exist for pain relief.

BREAST-FEEDING: This drug is found in breast milk. The American Academy of Pediatrics considers this drug to be compatible with breast-feeding. As with all drugs, some caution should still be used.

BRAND NAME: **Nasacort**

GENERIC NAME: **Triamcinolone acetonide**

USES: **To treat nasal allergies**

FDA PREGNANCY CATEGORY: **C**

VIRTUALLY NO RISK	SLIGHT RISK	MODERATE RISK	STRONG RISK	EXTREME RISK

Nasacort is a steroid that is inhaled through the nose to treat allergies and runny nose. Inhaled triamcinolone has been found to cause birth defects in monkeys at doses 18 times the recommended human dose. Adverse effects that were observed include deformities in the brain and skull. There are no studies concerning the use of Nasacort in pregnant women. Nasacort should not be used in pregnancy unless its benefits outweigh its risks to the fetus.

BREAST-FEEDING: It is not known whether the drug is found in breast milk. Caution should be used when breast-feeding.

BRAND NAME: **Nasonex**

GENERIC NAME: **mometasone furoate**

USES: **To treat nasal allergies**

FDA PREGNANCY CATEGORY: **C**

VIRTUALLY NO RISK	SLIGHT RISK	MODERATE RISK	STRONG RISK	EXTREME RISK

Nasonex is a steroid spray inhaled through the nose to treat allergies and runny nose. Nasonex has been found to cause birth defects in rabbits given 14 times the normal human dose, and in rats given up to 30 times the normal human dose. Some of the birth defects that were observed include hernias, slowed bone development, and cleft palate. No studies have been conducted assessing the use of Nasonex during human pregnancy. It is not recommended for use during pregnancy.

BREAST-FEEDING: It is not known whether the drug is found in breast milk. Caution should be used when breast-feeding.

BRAND NAME: **Natalins Rx**
GENERIC NAME: **prenatal multivitamin**
USES: **As a nutritional supplement during pregnancy and breast-feeding**
FDA PREGNANCY CATEGORY: **B**

VIRTUALLY NO RISK	SLIGHT RISK	MODERATE RISK	STRONG RISK	EXTREME RISK
▨				

Multiple vitamin supplements are routinely given to pregnant women since vitamins are needed for a healthy baby. The use of multivitamins up to the recommended daily allowance is suggested during pregnancy for the general health of the mother and fetus. There is evidence that proper supplementation, especially with folic acid, can reduce the risk of cleft palate and neural tube defects such as spina bifida. Use of a multivitamin during pregnancy is highly recommended under the supervision of a physician.

BREAST-FEEDING: This drug is found in breast milk. The American Academy of Pediatrics considers this drug to be compatible with breast-feeding.

BRAND NAME: **Neurontin**
GENERIC NAME: **gabapentin**
USES: **To treat epilepsy and seizures**
FDA PREGNANCY CATEGORY: **C**

VIRTUALLY NO RISK	SLIGHT RISK	MODERATE RISK	STRONG RISK	EXTREME RISK
▨	▨	▨		

Only two reports exist regarding the use of this drug during pregnancy. No concrete links can be made to Neurontin causing the birth defects.

The lack of data regarding the use of this drug during pregnancy does not allow a conclusion to be made regarding its safety. The potential benefit would have to significantly outweigh the potential risk to the fetus before choosing to use this drug.

BREAST-FEEDING: It is not known whether the drug is found in breast milk. Extreme caution should be used when breast-feeding.

BRAND NAME: **Nizoral**
GENERIC NAME: **ketoconazole**
USES: **To treat fungal infections**
FDA PREGNANCY CATEGORY: **C**

VIRTUALLY NO RISK	SLIGHT RISK	MODERATE RISK	STRONG RISK	EXTREME RISK

Nizoral is an antifungal agent that is usually not recommended for use in pregnancy. This drug has been found to be toxic to the embryo and to cause birth defects as well. In an observational study, 20 newborns had been exposed to oral Nizoral during the first trimester and none of the infants showed any birth defects. However, the FDA has started to receive reports of defects in the arms and legs of infants who had been exposed to Nizoral during pregnancy. The use of Nizoral is not recommended during pregnancy unless its benefits strongly outweigh its potential risks to the fetus.

BREAST-FEEDING: This drug is found in breast milk. The potential effects of exposure to this drug on a breast-feeding infant are not known. Nursing mothers taking this drug should use caution when breast-feeding.

BRAND NAME: **Nolvadex**

GENERIC NAME: **tamoxifen**

USES: **Cancer (primarily breast cancer)**

FDA PREGNANCY CATEGORY: **D**

VIRTUALLY NO RISK	SLIGHT RISK	MODERATE RISK	STRONG RISK	EXTREME RISK

Tamoxifen is known to produce toxic changes in the reproductive tract of animals, with similar effects seen in humans. In addition, a number of fetal and neonatal defects have been reported, including malformations in the genitalia. Tamoxifen could also cause developmental abnormalities of the genital tract in children later in life. An increased incidence of miscarriages is also a possibility. This drug should be avoided if at all possible at least eight weeks prior to pregnancy and throughout pregnancy to prevent the potential harm to the fetus.

BREAST-FEEDING: This drug is found in breast milk and may be harmful to a breast-feeding infant. This drug should not be taken by nursing mothers.

BRAND NAME: **Norflex**

GENERIC NAME: **orphenadrine**

USES: **To treat muscle spasms**

FDA PREGNANCY CATEGORY: **C**

VIRTUALLY NO RISK	SLIGHT RISK	MODERATE RISK	STRONG RISK	EXTREME RISK

There are no clinical studies regarding the use of Norflex during pregnancy. When given to rats in large doses, it has been found to cause enlarged bladders. With the lack of information available, the potential benefit to the mother must very significantly outweigh the potential risk to the fetus for Norflex to be prescribed.

BREAST-FEEDING: It is not known whether the drug is found in breast milk. Caution should be used when breast-feeding.

BRAND NAME: **Norvasc**
GENERIC NAME: **amlodipine**
USES: **To treat high blood pressure and angina**
FDA PREGNANCY CATEGORY: **C**

VIRTUALLY NO RISK	SLIGHT RISK	MODERATE RISK	STRONG RISK	EXTREME RISK

This drug of the calcium channel blocker family has not been studied in pregnant women. However, rats and rabbits were given a single dose up to 8 to 10 times the normal dose. At these doses, no birth defects were shown. When rats were given 8 times the recommended human dose for two weeks, the results were a decrease in litter size and prolonged labor and gestation. With the possibility of risk to the fetus, Norvasc should be used with caution.

BREAST-FEEDING: It is not known whether the drug is found in breast milk. Caution should be used when breast-feeding.

BRAND NAME: **Ortho-Cept**
GENERIC NAME: **Combination product containing desogestrel and ethinyl estradiol**
Similar to **Alesse-28;** see entry for **Alesse-28**

BRAND NAME: **Ortho-Cyclen**
GENERIC NAME: **Combination product containing norgestimate and ethinyl estradiol**
Similar to **Alesse-28;** see entry for **Alesse-28**

BRAND NAME: **Ortho-Novum 7/7/7**

GENERIC NAME: **Combination product containing norethindrone and ethinyl estradiol**

Similar to **Alesse-28**; see entry for **Alesse-28**

BRAND NAME: **Ortho Tri-Cyclen**

GENERIC NAME: **Combination product containing norgestimate and ethinyl estradiol**

Similar to **Alesse-28**; see entry for **Alesse-28**

BRAND NAME: **Pamelor**

GENERIC NAME: **nortriptyline**

USES: **To treat depression and insomnia**

FDA PREGNANCY CATEGORY: **C**

VIRTUALLY NO RISK	SLIGHT RISK	MODERATE RISK	STRONG RISK	EXTREME RISK

There are limited reports regarding the use of Pamelor during pregnancy. Limb malformations have been noted; however, no clear connection can be made between the drug and the defects. Bladder problems have also been associated with the drug when used during pregnancy. With minimal information available, this drug should be used with caution and only if absolutely necessary.

BREAST-FEEDING: This drug is found in breast milk and may be harmful to a breast-feeding infant. This drug should not be taken by nursing mothers.

BRAND NAME: **Paxil**

GENERIC NAME: **paroxetine**

USES: **To treat depression, panic disorder, and obessive-compulsive disorder**

FDA PREGNANCY CATEGORY: **B**

VIRTUALLY NO RISK	SLIGHT RISK	MODERATE RISK	STRONG RISK	EXTREME RISK
▮				

Paxil is a drug used to treat depression by interacting with a chemical in the brain known as serotonin. Studies in rats given doses up to 50 times the maximum recommended human daily doses showed no developmental abnormalities. In a study conducted after Paxil came on the market, no abnormalities were noted in infants born to mothers who had taken the drug. The small amount of data concerning the safety of Paxil and pregnancy should limit the use until further studies are done to prove its safety. Currently, Prozac is considered a better choice.

BREAST-FEEDING: This drug is found in breast milk. The potential effects of exposure to this drug on a breast-feeding infant are not known. Nursing mothers taking this drug should use caution when breast-feeding.

BRAND NAME: **PCE**

GENERIC NAME: **erythromycin**

See entry for **E-mycin**

BRAND NAME: **Pentasa**

GENERIC NAME: **mesalamine**

USES: **To treat mildly to moderately active ulcerative colitis**

FDA PREGNANCY CATEGORY: **B**

VIRTUALLY NO RISK	SLIGHT RISK	MODERATE RISK	STRONG RISK	EXTREME RISK
▮	▮			

Pentasa is an oral drug used to treat inflammatory bowel disorders. In animal studies, rats were given doses up to 1000mg/kg/day and rabbits were given doses up to 800mg/kg/day, and no evidence of birth defects was shown. Although Pentasa is known to cross the placenta, there have been no adequate studies looking at the effects of Pentasa use during pregnancy. The benefits of using this drug during pregnancy usually outweigh the potential risks to the fetus.

BREAST-FEEDING: This drug is found in breast milk and may be harmful to a breast-feeding infant. This drug should not be taken by nursing mothers.

BRAND NAME: **Pepcid**
GENERIC NAME: **famotidine**
USES: **To treat active stomach ulcers, active duodenal ulcers (ulcers of the upper part of the small intestine, also called peptic ulcers), for maintenance of healed duodenal ulcers, and for the treatment of gastroesophageal reflux disease (GERD)**
FDA PREGNANCY CATEGORY: **B**

VIRTUALLY NO RISK	SLIGHT RISK	MODERATE RISK	STRONG RISK	EXTREME RISK

There are no clinical studies regarding the use of this drug during pregnancy. However, in studies on rats and rabbits, high doses have been given during pregnancy and no evidence of birth defects or infertility has been reported. But at 250 times the human dose in rabbits, abortions have been noted. With limited experience on the use of Pepcid during pregnancy in humans, this drug should be used with some caution during pregnancy.

BREAST-FEEDING: This drug is found in breast milk. The potential effects of exposure to this drug on a breast-feeding infant are not known. Nursing mothers taking this drug should use some caution when breast-feeding.

BRAND NAME: **Percocet**

GENERIC NAME: **Combination product containing acetaminophen and oxycodone**

USES: **To treat moderate to severe pain**

FDA PREGNANCY CATEGORY: **C**

VIRTUALLY NO RISK	SLIGHT RISK	MODERATE RISK	STRONG RISK	EXTREME RISK

The acetaminophen component of this drug is safe to use during all stages of pregnancy. Acetaminophen should only be used for short periods of time, because long-term use can cause problems in the infant, such as anemia or low red blood cell count. However, because of the oxycodone component some caution is needed. Minor malformations have been found, but they could not definitely be linked to this drug. One study looked at first-trimester exposure and found no evidence of birth defects. The oxycodone component of this drug can cause withdrawal in infants if mothers use high doses. If used for prolonged periods or in high doses, this drug becomes more risky. This drug should be used with extreme caution if used for long periods of time during pregnancy.

BREAST-FEEDING: This drug is found in breast milk. The potential effects of exposure to this drug on a breast-feeding infant are not known. Nursing mothers taking this drug should use extreme caution when breast-feeding.

BRAND NAME: **Phenergan**

GENERIC NAME: **promethazine**

USES: **To treat allergies, allergic reactions, cough, nausea, vomiting, and motion sickness**

FDA PREGNANCY CATEGORY: **C**

VIRTUALLY NO RISK	SLIGHT RISK	MODERATE RISK	STRONG RISK	EXTREME RISK

Phenergan is a drug most commonly used to treat nausea and vomiting. Across numerous studies, there has been little evidence that linked Phenergan to adverse effects in the fetus. However, in a large study in Michigan, a small percentage of infants had adverse effects after being exposed to Phenergan in the first trimester, with cardiovascular defects being the most common. Other factors, including disease in the mother and use of other drugs, could have also contributed to these birth defects. When given to the mother near delivery, difficulty breathing has been noticed in the infants, as well as a possible increased risk for bleeding. Phenergan should not be used during pregnancy unless its benefits outweigh the risks to the fetus.

BREAST-FEEDING: This drug is found in breast milk. The potential effects of exposure to this drug on a breast-feeding infant are not known. Nursing mothers taking this drug should use caution when breast-feeding.

BRAND NAME: **Phrenilin**

GENERIC NAME: **Combination product containing butalbital and acetaminophen**

USES: **To treat tension headache**

FDA PREGNANCY CATEGORY: **C**

VIRTUALLY NO RISK	SLIGHT RISK	MODERATE RISK	STRONG RISK	EXTREME RISK

Phrenelin is a combination of two ingredients, bultalbital and acetaminophen (Tylenol®). Butalbital is a barbiturate drug usually used to treat pain. No adequate studies have been conducted in animals to determine if butalbital causes birth defects. In one human study, a small percentage of birth defects, including cardiovascular defects and spina bifida, was reported. In 112 newborns exposed to butalbital during the first trimester, there were no malformations reported. Butalbital should not be considered for long-term use or in high doses near the end of pregnancy. Acetaminophen (Tylenol®) is generally considered safe for use during all trimesters of pregnancy for short-term pain relief and fever reduction. Unlike aspirin, acetaminophen does not interfere with platelet function and therefore does not cause a problem with bleeding when given near delivery. This combination product is not recommended during pregnancy unless its potential benefits outweigh the risks involved.

BREAST-FEEDING: It is not known whether the drug is found in breast milk. Caution should be used when breast-feeding.

BRAND NAME: **Plendil**
GENERIC NAME: **felodipine**
USES: **To treat high blood pressure**
FDA PREGNANCY CATEGORY: **C**

VIRTUALLY NO RISK	SLIGHT RISK	MODERATE RISK	STRONG RISK	EXTREME RISK

Minor defects have been noted with the use of this drug during pregnancy. In rabbits and rats, fingers formed incorrectly were found. At four times the maximum human dose, mothers experienced difficult labors, increased number of stillbirths, and decreased incidence of survival after delivery. In addition, three cases of pregnant mothers using this drug reported no adverse effects to the fetus. However, one of the three births was preterm with a low-birthweight newborn. With the potential risks associated with the use of this drug during pregnancy, other options should be considered first.

BREAST-FEEDING: This drug is found in breast milk. The potential effects of exposure to this drug on a breast-feeding infant are not known. Women taking this drug should use caution when breast-feeding.

BRAND NAME: **Pravachol**

GENERIC NAME: **pravastatin**

Similar to **Mevacor;** see entry for **Mevacor**

BRAND NAME: **Precose**

GENERIC NAME: **acarbose**

USES: **To treat diabetes**

FDA PREGNANCY CATEGORY: **B**

VIRTUALLY NO RISK	SLIGHT RISK	MODERATE RISK	STRONG RISK	EXTREME RISK

Precose is a drug used to control blood sugar in patients who have diabetes. Precose is usually not a drug of first choice during pregnancy. Although only 2 percent of a dose is absorbed into the bloodstream, the body has the ability to change this drug into a different compounds and these products could be harmful to the fetus. Doses of up to 32 times the normal human dose were given to rabbits and no birth defects were reported. No reports are currently available concerning the use of Precose in human pregnancy. Precose should not be used to control blood sugar in patients who are pregnant and have diabetes. Insulin is the drug of choice for all pregnant diabetic patients.

BREAST-FEEDING: This drug is found in breast milk. The potential effects of exposure to this drug on a breast-feeding infant are not known. Nursing mothers taking this drug should use caution when breast-feeding.

BRAND NAME: **Prednisone**

GENERIC NAME: **prednisone**

USES: **To treat inflammation and immune system problems**

FDA PREGNANCY CATEGORY: **B**

VIRTUALLY NO RISK	SLIGHT RISK	MODERATE RISK	STRONG RISK	EXTREME RISK

Prednisone is a corticosteroid used to treat many diseases and is thought to have only a small effect on the developing fetus. One instance of cataracts in an infant exposed to prednisone has been reported. Prednisone is used to help premature infants who are having trouble breathing. The use of prednisone in pregnancy should be considered when the beneficial effects of controlling a mother's problem outweigh the risks to the fetus.

BREAST-FEEDING: This drug is found in breast milk. The potential effects of exposure to this drug on a breast-feeding infant are not known. Nursing mothers taking this drug should use caution when breast-feeding.

BRAND NAME: **Prenate Ultra**
GENERIC NAME: **prenatal vitamin with docusate sodium**
USES: **As a nutritional supplement during pregnancy and breast-feeding**
FDA PREGNANCY CATEGORY: **B**

VIRTUALLY NO RISK	SLIGHT RISK	MODERATE RISK	STRONG RISK	EXTREME RISK

Multiple vitamin supplements are routinely given to pregnant women since vitamins are needed for a healthy baby. The use of multivitamins up to the recommended daily allowance is recommended during pregnancy for the general health of the mother and fetus. There is evidence that proper supplementation, especially with folic acid, can reduce the risk for cleft palate and neural tube defects such as spina bifida. Use of a multivitamin during pregnancy is highly recommended under the supervision of a physician.

BREAST-FEEDING: This drug is found in breast milk. However, the American Academy of Pediatrics considers this drug to be compatible with breast-feeding.

BRAND NAME: **Prevacid**

GENERIC NAME: **lansoprazole**

USES: **To treat ulcers, gastroesophageal reflux disease (GERD), and Zollinger-Ellison syndrome**

FDA PREGNANCY CATEGORY: **B**

VIRTUALLY NO RISK	SLIGHT RISK	MODERATE RISK	STRONG RISK	EXTREME RISK

This drug has not been studied in humans during pregnancy. However, when this drug was given to rats and rabbits at high doses, no evidence of harm to the fetus was reported. A decrease in fetal weight occurred in one study with no birth defects found. When another drug in the same class, Prilosec, was given to pregnant women, birth defects were reported. Some of these defects included deformed feet and missing brain or spinal cord, which led to fetal death. With these results noted for Prilosec and with no reports using this drug during human pregnancy, caution is advised. Until human studies are available, this drug should be used with extreme caution during pregnancy.

BREAST-FEEDING: This drug is found in breast milk and may be harmful to a breast-feeding infant. This drug should not be taken by nursing mothers.

BRAND NAME: **Prilosec**

GENERIC NAME: **omeprazole**

USES: **To treat ulcers, gastroesophageal reflux disease (GERD), and Zollinger-Ellison syndrome**

FDA PREGNANCY CATEGORY: **C**

VIRTUALLY NO RISK	SLIGHT RISK	MODERATE RISK	STRONG RISK	EXTREME RISK

When this drug was given to pregnant women, birth defects were reported. Some of these defects include deformed feet and missing brain or spinal cord, which led to fetal death. Considering these results, extreme caution should be taken by pregnant mothers. Until further data is available to assess the risk to the fetus, this drug should not be used during pregnancy, especially during the first trimester.

BREAST-FEEDING: This drug is found in breast milk and may be harmful to a breast-feeding infant. This drug should not be taken by nursing mothers.

BRAND NAME: **Prinivil**
GENERIC NAME: **lisinopril**
USES: **To treat high blood pressure and heart failure**
FDA PREGNANCY CATEGORY: **D**

VIRTUALLY NO RISK	SLIGHT RISK	MODERATE RISK	STRONG RISK	EXTREME RISK

Prinivil should be used only with extreme caution during pregnancy. In the second and third trimesters of pregnancy, it has been shown to cause severe birth defects and possible death of the fetus. During the first trimester of pregnancy, its safety is only slightly better. Prinivil should not be used at all during pregnancy unless all other therapeutic options have been exhausted.

BREAST-FEEDING: It is not known whether the drug is found in breast milk. Caution should be used when breast-feeding.

BRAND NAME: **Procardia XL**
GENERIC NAME: **nifedipine**
USES: **To treat angina and high blood pressure**
FDA PREGNANCY CATEGORY: **C**

VIRTUALLY NO RISK	SLIGHT RISK	MODERATE RISK	STRONG RISK	EXTREME RISK

Data regarding the use of Procardia XL during pregnancy is limited. In monkeys, minor birth defects have been seen, such as decreased oxygen available to the fetus. With this information and other animal studies in mind, this drug should be reserved for use in patients with severely high blood pressure who are unresponsive to standard, safer therapy. The toxicity of this drug may outweigh its potential benefits.

BREAST-FEEDING: This drug is found in breast milk. The potential effects of exposure to this drug on a breast-feeding infant are not known. Nursing mothers taking this drug should use caution when breast-feeding.

BRAND NAME: **ProSom**
GENERIC NAME: **estazolam**
USES: **To treat insomnia**
FDA PREGNANCY CATEGORY: **X**

VIRTUALLY NO RISK	SLIGHT RISK	MODERATE RISK	STRONG RISK	EXTREME RISK

ProSom is a benzodiazepine that is used in the treatment of insomnia. Under no circumstances should it be taken during pregnancy. Benzodiazepines have been associated with central nervous system depression, decreased breathing, and decreased heart rate in the fetus. This category of drugs has been associated with many fetal malformations, including cleft palate and birth defects in the fetal brain. Fetal withdrawal has been shown after delivery when the mother had been taking ProSom during pregnancy. ProSom is not to be taken during pregnancy for any reason because of the potential for adverse effects to the fetus.

BREAST-FEEDING: This drug is found in breast milk and may be harmful to a breast-feeding infant. This drug should not be taken by nursing mothers.

BRAND NAME: **Proventil**

GENERIC NAME: **albuterol**

USES: **To treat asthma, chronic bronchitis, emphysema, and other breathing disorders**

FDA PREGNANCY CATEGORY: **C**

VIRTUALLY NO RISK	SLIGHT RISK	MODERATE RISK	STRONG RISK	EXTREME RISK

Proventil is a drug that comes in oral and inhaled forms. The inhaled form of Proventil is used to treat asthma attacks. In one study, 12 pregnant women received two inhalations daily during their pregnancy and no adverse affects were reported. In another case, a patient was overdosed on inhaled Proventil and fetal heart rate increased rapidly. Proventil may also cause an increase in blood sugar for both the mother and the fetus. Oral Proventil has been used to prevent early labor. In an observational study, a small percentage of infants exposed to Proventil during the first trimester had major birth defects, with an increased number of fingers/toes being a common defect. Proventil should only be used in pregnancy when the benefits strongly outweigh the risks to the fetus.

BREAST-FEEDING: It is not known whether the drug is found in breast milk. Caution should be used when breast-feeding.

BRAND NAME: **Prozac**

GENERIC NAME: **fluoxetine**

USES: **To treat depression, bulimia, and obsessive-compulsive disorder**

FDA PREGNANCY CATEGORY: **B**

VIRTUALLY NO RISK	SLIGHT RISK	MODERATE RISK	STRONG RISK	EXTREME RISK

Many studies have been done on the use of Prozac during pregnancy and an increase risk of minor defects has been observed. If taken during the third trimester, there is an increased risk of low birth weight and complications with the breathing of the fetus. These effects appear to be relatively minor. It was also found that Prozac does not affect the future development of the children who were exposed to this drug during pregnancy. With no concrete evidence of this drug causing major problems, this drug may be used with some caution during pregnancy if its benefits outweigh the risks.

BREAST-FEEDING: This drug is found in breast milk and may be harmful to a breast-feeding infant. This drug should not be taken by nursing mothers.

BRAND NAME: **Pyridium**
GENERIC NAME: **phenazopyridine**
USES: **To provide relief of pain, burning, urgency, frequency, and other symptoms associated with a urinary tract infection**
FDA PREGNANCY CATEGORY: **B**

VIRTUALLY NO RISK	SLIGHT RISK	MODERATE RISK	STRONG RISK	EXTREME RISK

There are no reports of birth defects associated with this drug. Hernias were a minor adverse effect reported in one study. The risk of malformations due to first-trimester exposure to this drug appears to be small. With minimal data available, however, some caution should be used when taking this drug during pregnancy.

BREAST-FEEDING: It is not known whether the drug is found in breast milk. Some caution should be used when breast-feeding.

BRAND NAME: **Reglan**

GENERIC NAME: **metoclopramide**

USES: **To treat nausea, vomiting, and gastroesophogeal reflux disease (GERD)**

FDA PREGNANCY CATEGORY: **B**

VIRTUALLY NO RISK	SLIGHT RISK	MODERATE RISK	STRONG RISK	EXTREME RISK
░░░░	░░░░			

Reglan is a drug used to treat various stomach and intestinal problems. Studies performed on rats, mice, and rabbits at doses ranging from 12 to 250 times the human dose have shown no significant harm to the fetus. There are no studies on the use of Reglan in pregnant women. Because of the lack of safety data, Reglan should be used with caution during pregnancy.

BREAST-FEEDING: Reglan is found in breast milk and may be harmful to a breast-feeding infant. It should not be taken by nursing mothers.

BRAND NAME: **Relafen**

GENERIC NAME: **nabumetone**

USES: **For arthritis and pain relief**

FDA PREGNANCY CATEGORY: **C**

VIRTUALLY NO RISK	SLIGHT RISK	MODERATE RISK	STRONG RISK	EXTREME RISK
░░░░	░░░░	░░░░		

There are no clinical studies on the use of Relafen during pregnancy. In animal studies, fetal toxicities have been minimal; they include decreased fetal growth and lengthened delivery. If this drug is used in the third trimester, abnormally high blood pressure has been found in the lungs of some infants. Also, Relafen should be avoided in those trying to conceive because it can block implantation of the fertilized egg. When used near delivery or in the third trimester, this drug is classified as a strong risk because of the possible increase in blood pressure in the lungs of the fetus. It has also been shown to prolong pregnancies and slow down labor. Relafen only should be used with extreme caution during pregnancy.

BREAST-FEEDING: It is not known whether the drug is found in breast milk. Caution should be used when breast-feeding.

BRAND NAME: **Remeron**
GENERIC NAME: **mirtazapine**
USES: **To treat depression**
FDA PREGNANCY CATEGORY: **C**

VIRTUALLY NO RISK	SLIGHT RISK	MODERATE RISK	STRONG RISK	EXTREME RISK

Remeron is a drug used to treat depression and has not been studied in human pregnancy. Rats given doses greater than 100mg, 17 times the maximum recommended human dose, showed no developmental abnormalities in the fetus. It is unknown whether Remeron crosses the placenta. The use of this drug is not recommended during pregnancy.

BREAST-FEEDING: It is not known whether the drug is found in breast milk. Caution should be used when breast-feeding.

BRAND NAME: **Restoril**
GENERIC NAME: **temazepam**
USES: **To treat insomnia**
FDA PREGNANCY CATEGORY: **X**

VIRTUALLY NO RISK	SLIGHT RISK	MODERATE RISK	STRONG RISK	EXTREME RISK

When this drug was administered to rats, birth defects were observed. But no definitive reports have been found linking this drug to birth defects in humans. Restoril is a benzodiazepine used in the treatment of insomnia, and under no circumstances should it be taken during pregnancy. Benzodiazepines have been associated with central nervous system depression, decreased breathing, and decreased heart rate in the fetus. This category of drugs has been associated with many fetal malformations, including cleft palate and birth defects in the brain. Fetal withdrawal has been shown after delivery when the mother had been taking Restoril during pregnancy. As stated above, Restoril should never be taken during pregnancy for any reason because of the potential for adverse effects in the fetus.

BREAST-FEEDING: This drug is found in breast milk. The potential effects of exposure to this drug on a breast-feeding infant are not known. Nursing mothers taking this drug should use extreme caution when breast-feeding.

BRAND NAME: **Retin-A**
GENERIC NAME: **tretinoin**
USES: **To treat acne**
FDA PREGNANCY CATEGORY: **C**

VIRTUALLY NO RISK	SLIGHT RISK	MODERATE RISK	STRONG RISK	EXTREME RISK

Topical Retin-A is not recommended for use during pregnancy due to the many birth defects linked to the drug's use. Even though the drug is applied to the skin, the drug is absorbed into the bloodstream and can cause serious birth defects, including facial deformities, cardiovascular and central nervous system defects, and abnormalities in male reproductive organs.

BREAST-FEEDING: It is not known whether the drug is found in breast milk. However, due to the possibility of serious adverse effects, extreme caution should be used when breast-feeding.

BRAND NAME: **Rhinocort**

GENERIC NAME: **budesonide**

USES: **To treat nasal allergies**

FDA PREGNANCY CATEGORY: **C**

VIRTUALLY NO RISK	SLIGHT RISK	MODERATE RISK	STRONG RISK	EXTREME RISK
▨	▨	▨		

Rhinocort is a steroid inhaled through the nose that is used in the treatment of allergies and runny nose. When rats and rabbits were given shots of budesonide, decreased weight of the fetus, malformations in the skeleton, and even fetal death occurred. However, when the animals were given inhaled doses of budesonide up to 68 times the normal human dose, no birth defects were observed. There are no studies dealing with the use of Rhinocort in pregnant women. Rhinocort is not recommended for use during pregnancy.

BREAST-FEEDING: This drug is found in breast milk. The potential effects of exposure to this drug on a breast-feeding infant are not known. Nursing mothers taking this drug should use caution when breast-feeding.

BRAND NAME: **Risperdal**

GENERIC NAME: **risperidone**

USES: **To treat psychotic disorders**

FDA PREGNANCY CATEGORY: **C**

VIRTUALLY NO RISK	SLIGHT RISK	MODERATE RISK	STRONG RISK	EXTREME RISK
▨	▨	▨		

When Risperdal was studied in rats and rabbits, an increase in birth defects was not seen; however, birth defects in the fetus have been reported. Death in animal fetuses was reported at 1.5 times the human dose. It is not known how this drug affects the mother or the fetus during human pregnancy. One case reported an infant missing part of his brain at birth. Since there are no adequate studies dealing with the use

of this drug during pregnancy, Risperdal should only be used if its benefits to the mother justify the possible risks to the fetus.

BREAST-FEEDING: It is not known whether the drug is found in breast milk.
Extreme caution should be used when breast-feeding.

BRAND NAME: **Ritalin**

GENERIC NAME: **methylphenidate**

USES: **To treat attention deficit disorders with hyperactivity (ADDH) in
children six years and older, and narcolepsy in adults**

FDA PREGNANCY CATEGORY: **C**

VIRTUALLY NO RISK	SLIGHT RISK	MODERATE RISK	STRONG RISK	EXTREME RISK

Adequate studies have not been performed to establish the safety of
this drug during pregnancy. In one study, no birth defects were reported. In another study, premature delivery, stunted growth, and withdrawal symptoms after delivery were observed. However, other drugs
were taken by the participants in this study and no direct link to Ritalin
can be made. To justify the use of this drug during pregnancy, the benefits to the mother must clearly outweigh the risks to the fetus.

BREAST-FEEDING: This drug may be found in breast milk and could be dangerous. However, the potential effects of exposure to this drug on a
breast-feeding infant are not known. Nursing mothers taking this drug
should use extreme caution when breast-feeding.

BRAND NAME: **Serax**

GENERIC NAME: **oxazepam**

USES: **To treat anxiety and alcohol withdrawal**

FDA PREGNANCY CATEGORY: **D**

VIRTUALLY NO RISK	SLIGHT RISK	MODERATE RISK	STRONG RISK	EXTREME RISK

Serax is a benzodiazepine used to treat anxiety and sleeping problems. Serax easily crosses the placenta and concentrates in the fetus. After exposure to Serax during pregnancy, adverse effects to the fetus such as growth retardation, abnormal features, central nervous system disorders, and mental retardation have been reported. Therefore, Serax should not be used during pregnancy.

BREAST-FEEDING: This drug is found in breast milk and may be harmful to a breast-feeding infant. This drug should not be taken by nursing mothers.

BRAND NAME: **Serevent**

GENERIC NAME: **salmeterol**

USES: **To treat asthma and other breathing disorders**

FDA PREGNANCY CATEGORY: **C**

VIRTUALLY NO RISK	SLIGHT RISK	MODERATE RISK	STRONG RISK	EXTREME RISK

Serevent is a long-acting inhaled drug used to treat asthma. In studies done in rabbits, oral doses up to 20 times the maximum recommended human dose caused numerous birth defects, including cleft palate, abnormal bone growth, and delayed hardening of bones in the skull. Studies have not been conducted examining the use of Serevent in pregnant women. Serevent is not recommended for use during pregnancy unless its benefits outweigh its potential risks to the fetus.

BREAST-FEEDING: It is not known whether the drug is found in breast milk. Caution should be used when breast-feeding.

BRAND NAME: **Seroquel**
GENERIC NAME: **quetiapine**
USES: **To treat psychosis**
FDA PREGNANCY CATEGORY: **C**

VIRTUALLY NO RISK	SLIGHT RISK	MODERATE RISK	STRONG RISK	EXTREME RISK
▨	▨	▨		

When this drug was studied in rats and rabbits, no birth defects were documented. However, the drug may cause some minor adverse effects in the fetus during pregnancy. Some of these adverse effects include delays in bone development and reduced body weight. At three times the maximum dose, increases in fetal death were reported. It is not known how this drug affects the mother or the fetus during a human pregnancy. Since there are no adequate studies regarding its use, Seroquel should only be used if its benefits to the mother justify the possible risks to the fetus.

BREAST-FEEDING: This drug is found in breast milk and may be harmful to a breast-feeding infant. This drug should not be taken by nursing mothers.

BRAND NAME: **Serzone**
GENERIC NAME: **nefazodone**
USES: **To treat depression**
FDA PREGNANCY CATEGORY: **C**

VIRTUALLY NO RISK	SLIGHT RISK	MODERATE RISK	STRONG RISK	EXTREME RISK
▨	▨	▨		

When Serzone was studied in rats and rabbits, no birth defects were reported. Currently, there are no reports regarding the use of this drug during human pregnancy. Because minimal data is available, another drug, such as Prozac, may be a better option if treatment for depression is necessary. Serzone should be used with caution during pregnancy.

BREAST-FEEDING: This drug is found in breast milk. The potential effects of exposure to this drug on a breast-feeding infant are not known. Nursing mothers taking this drug should use caution when breast-feeding.

BRAND NAME: **Skelaxin**
GENERIC NAME: **metaxalone**
USES: **To treat muscle spasms**
FDA PREGNANCY CATEGORY: **None established**

VIRTUALLY NO RISK	SLIGHT RISK	MODERATE RISK	STRONG RISK	EXTREME RISK

In studies on rats, this drug caused no harm to the fetus, but no reports of the use of this drug in humans has been reported. The safety of Skelaxin during pregnancy has not been established and the potential for adverse affects on the fetus is real. This drug should not be used by pregnant women unless the benefits outweigh the possible harm to the fetus.

BREAST-FEEDING: It is not known whether the drug is found in breast milk. Caution should be used when breast-feeding.

BRAND NAME: **Slo-bid**
GENERIC NAME: **theophylline**
USES: **To treat asthma, chronic bronchitis, emphysema, and other breathing disorders**
FDA PREGNANCY CATEGORY: **C**

VIRTUALLY NO RISK	SLIGHT RISK	MODERATE RISK	STRONG RISK	EXTREME RISK

Slo-bid is used to treat asthma and other breathing disorders. It crosses the placenta and has been associated with birth defects, including cardiovascular problems, oral clefts, and spina bifida. In mothers using Slo-bid, increased heart rate, irritability, and vomiting have been seen in newborns after delivery. Slo-bid should be used in pregnancy only if its benefits greatly outweigh its potential risks to the fetus.

BREAST-FEEDING: This drug is found in breast milk. The potential effects of exposure to this drug on a breast-feeding infant are not known. Women taking this drug should use extreme caution when breast-feeding.

BRAND NAME: **Soma**
GENERIC NAME: **carisoprodol**
USES: **As a muscle relaxer and painkiller**
FDA PREGNANCY CATEGORY: **C**

VIRTUALLY NO RISK	SLIGHT RISK	MODERATE RISK	STRONG RISK	EXTREME RISK
▓▓▓▓	▓▓▓▓	▓▓▓▓		

Soma is a product usually used as a muscle relaxant and to treat pain. It has not been studied in animal or human pregnancies. Soma should not be used during pregnancy because of the lack of any data, human or animal, and its potential risks during pregnancy.

BREAST-FEEDING: This drug is found in breast milk. The potential effects of exposure to this drug on a breast-feeding infant are not known. Nursing mothers taking this drug should use caution when breast-feeding.

BRAND NAME: **Sporanox**

GENERIC NAME: **itraconazole**

USES: **To treat fungal infections**

FDA PREGNANCY CATEGORY: **C**

VIRTUALLY NO RISK	SLIGHT RISK	MODERATE RISK	STRONG RISK	EXTREME RISK

Sporanox is an antifungal agent that is generally not recommended for use during pregnancy. In rats treated with doses up to 5 to 20 times the recommended human dose, birth defects, including skeletal deformities, were seen. There are no human studies on the use of Sporanox during pregnancy. However, the FDA has received several reports concerning malformation and defects in the arms/legs of infants exposed to the drug during pregnancy. Due to the lack of safety data, the use of Sporanox is not recommended during pregnancy.

BREAST-FEEDING: This drug is found in breast milk and may be harmful to a breast-feeding infant. This drug should not be taken by nursing mothers.

BRAND NAME: **Sumycin**

GENERIC NAME: **tetracycline**

Very similar to **Minocin;** see entry for **Minocin**

BRAND NAME: **Suprax**

GENERIC NAME: **cefixime**

USES: **To treat bacterial infections**

FDA PREGNANCY CATEGORY: **B**

VIRTUALLY NO RISK	SLIGHT RISK	MODERATE RISK	STRONG RISK	EXTREME RISK

Suprax is an oral antibiotic used to treat various bacterial infections, and is generally considered safe for use during pregnancy. In rats given up to 400 times the normal human dose, no birth defects were reported. No studies are available that report on the use of Suprax in human pregnancy.

BREAST-FEEDING: This drug is found in breast milk. The potential effects of exposure to this drug on a breast-feeding infant are not known. Nursing mothers taking this drug should use some caution when breast-feeding.

BRAND NAME: **Synthroid**

GENERIC NAME: **levothyroxine**

USES: **Thyroid replacement therapy**

FDA PREGNANCY CATEGORY: **A**

VIRTUALLY NO RISK	SLIGHT RISK	MODERATE RISK	STRONG RISK	EXTREME RISK

Synthroid is a natural thyroid hormone that is produced by both the mother and the fetus. Most research claims that very little of the drug crosses the placenta. In a large study looking at infants exposed to thyroid hormone during the first trimester, some cardiovascular problems and Down syndrome were reported. There were not enough cases to directly link these birth defects to the thyroid hormone. Mothers who do not have enough thyroid hormone have been shown to have poor pregnancy outcomes. Although data is not complete, the use of thyroid hormone in pregnant women seems to be relatively safe.

BREAST-FEEDING: This drug is found in breast milk. The potential effects of exposure to this drug on a breast-feeding infant are not known. Nursing mothers taking this drug should use some caution when breast-feeding.

BRAND NAME: **Tenormin**

GENERIC NAME: **atenolol**

Similar to **Lopressor;** see entry for **Lopressor**

BRAND NAME: **Tessalon**

GENERIC NAME: **benzonatate**

USES: **To treat coughs**

FDA PREGNANCY CATEGORY: **C**

VIRTUALLY NO RISK	SLIGHT RISK	MODERATE RISK	STRONG RISK	EXTREME RISK

It is not known whether this drug causes harm to the fetus. There have been no studies on this drug in animals or humans. Tessalon should be used in pregnant women only if its benefits significantly outweigh its potential to harm the fetus.

BREAST-FEEDING: It is not known whether the drug is found in breast milk. Caution should be used when breast-feeding.

BRAND NAME: **Theo-Dur**

GENERIC NAME: **theophylline anhydrous**

Very similar to **Slo-bid;** see entry for **Slo-bid**

BRAND NAME: **Tigan**

GENERIC NAME: **trimethobenzamide**

USES: **To treat nausea and vomiting**

FDA PREGNANCY CATEGORY: **C**

VIRTUALLY NO RISK	SLIGHT RISK	MODERATE RISK	STRONG RISK	EXTREME RISK

Tigan is a drug that has been used to treat nausea and vomiting during pregnancy. When studied in pregnant women, there was a higher incidence of birth defects in the group that had received Tigan. However, it is unknown if the mother's disease or use of other drugs could have caused the defects as well. The use of Tigan is not recommended during pregnancy unless its benefits strongly outweigh its potential risks to the fetus.

BREAST-FEEDING: It is not known whether the drug is found in breast milk. Caution should be used when breast-feeding.

BRAND NAME: **Tilade**
GENERIC NAME: **nedocromil**
USES: **To treat asthma**
FDA PREGNANCY CATEGORY: **B**

VIRTUALLY NO RISK	SLIGHT RISK	MODERATE RISK	STRONG RISK	EXTREME RISK

Tilade is an inhaled drug used for maintenance therapy in mild to moderate asthma. Fetuses of rats given shots of Tilade at up to 60 times the normal human dose showed no adverse effects. There are no studies looking at the use of Tilade during pregnancy. Tilade, therefore, should be used with some caution during pregnancy.

BREAST-FEEDING: It is not known whether the drug is found in breast milk. Some caution should be used when breast-feeding.

BRAND NAME: **Tobradex**

GENERIC NAME: **tobramycin and dexamethasone**

USES: **To treat bacterial eye infections**

FDA PREGNANCY CATEGORY: **C**

VIRTUALLY NO RISK	SLIGHT RISK	MODERATE RISK	STRONG RISK	EXTREME RISK
▨	▨	▨		

Tobradex is a product containing two ingredients that is used to treat eye infections. The dexamethasone component is a steroid. In one study, administration of it into the eyes of pregnant rabbits resulted in a 32.3 percent rate of fetal abnormalities. Delayed growth and increased death have been observed in offspring of rats treated with long-term steroids. Tobramycin has been studied in rats at doses greater than 100mg and has not shown any harm to the fetus. No studies have been conducted in human pregnancy to evaluate the safety of this product. Tobradex is not recommended for use during pregnancy unless its benefits strongly outweigh its potential risks to the fetus.

BREAST-FEEDING: It is not known whether the drug is found in breast milk. Caution should be used when breast-feeding.

BRAND NAME: **Tofranil**

GENERIC NAME: **imipramine**

USES: **To treat depression and bedwetting**

FDA PREGNANCY CATEGORY: **D**

VIRTUALLY NO RISK	SLIGHT RISK	MODERATE RISK	STRONG RISK	EXTREME RISK
▨	▨	▨	▨	

Birth defects have been reported when this drug is used during pregnancy. Some of the reported defects include hernia, cleft palate, and defective muscle formation. Also, several infants have developed respiratory problems, jerky movements, increased respiratory rate, and convulsions shortly after birth. Tofranil should not be used during pregnancy.

BREAST-FEEDING: This drug is found in breast milk. The potential effects of exposure to this drug on a breast-feeding infant are not known. Nursing mothers taking this drug should use extreme caution when breast-feeding.

BRAND NAME: **Toprol XL**
GENERIC NAME: **metoprolol**
Similar to **Lopressor;** see entry for **Lopressor**

BRAND NAME: **Tranxene**
GENERIC NAME: **clorazepate**
USES: **To treat anxiety**
FDA PREGNANCY CATEGORY: **D**

VIRTUALLY NO RISK	SLIGHT RISK	MODERATE RISK	STRONG RISK	EXTREME RISK

Tranxene is a benzodiazepine and is therefore not recommended for use during pregnancy. No reports of malformation resulted when animals were given large doses. However, numerous reports from humans describe many abnormalities with the use of Tranxene and other benzodiazepines. Some of these deformities include abnormal fingers/toes, no scrotum or anus, cardiovascular defects, and the presence of more than one spleen in the infant. The use of Tranxene and other benzodiazepines is not recommended during pregnancy due to the serious birth defects that could result.

BREAST-FEEDING: It is not known whether the drug is found in breast milk. Extreme caution should be used when breast-feeding.

BRAND NAME: **Tri-Levlen**

GENERIC NAME: **Combination product containing levonorgestrel and ethinyl estradiol**

Similar to **Alesse-28;** see entry for **Alesse-28**

BRAND NAME: **Trimox**

GENERIC NAME: **amoxicillin**

Similar to **Amoxil;** see entry for **Amoxil**

BRAND NAME: **Trinalin**

GENERIC NAME: **Combination product containing pseudoephedrine and azatadine**

USES: **To treat nasal allergies and congestion**

FDA PREGNANCY CATEGORY: **C**

VIRTUALLY NO RISK	SLIGHT RISK	MODERATE RISK	STRONG RISK	EXTREME RISK

Trinalin is a drug that is composed of two ingredients—pseudoephedrine and azatadine. Pseudoephedrine, and other drugs in this same category, has been shown to cause birth defects in animals. Human studies in which first-trimester exposure to pseudoephedrine is reported have shown a significantly increased risk of fetal malformations. Many physicians suggest avoiding pseudoephedrine during the first trimester of pregnancy and to use some caution during the second and third trimesters. Azatadine has not been shown to cause developmental abnormalities in rats or rabbits, and no data on the use of azatadine in humans is available. One study reports a small percentage of birth defects in infants who were exposed to azatadine during the first trimester, including decreased number of arms or legs and an oral cleft. This product is not recommended for use during pregnancy unless its benefits outweigh its potential risks to the fetus.

BREAST-FEEDING: It is not known whether the drug is found in breast milk. Caution should be used when breast-feeding.

BRAND NAME: **Triphasil**
GENERIC NAME: **Combination product containing levonorgestrel and ethinyl estradiol**
Similar to **Alesse-28;** see entry for **Alesse-28**

BRAND NAME: **Tylenol No. 3**
GENERIC NAME: **Combination product containing acetaminophen and codeine**
USES: **To treat mild to moderate pain**
FDA PREGNANCY CATEGORY: **C**

VIRTUALLY NO RISK	SLIGHT RISK	MODERATE RISK	STRONG RISK	EXTREME RISK

Tylenol No. 3 contains two ingredients—acetaminophen and codeine. Acetaminophen (Tylenol) is generally considered safe for use during all trimesters of pregnancy for short-term pain relief and fever reduction. Unlike aspirin, acetaminophen does not interfere with platelet function and therefore does not cause a problem with bleeding when given near delivery. Codeine is a narcotic medication generally used to decrease pain. Codeine is not recommended for use in pregnancy because of its potential to cause abnormalities in the organs needed for breathing. Water on the brain, tumors, and hernias have been linked to the use of codeine. Because of the numerous possible adverse effects, this compound is not recommended for use during pregnancy unless absolutely necessary.

BREAST-FEEDING: This drug is found in breast milk. The potential effects of exposure to this drug on a breast-feeding infant are not known. Nursing mothers taking this drug should use extreme caution when breast-feeding.

BRAND NAME: **Ultram**

GENERIC NAME: **tramadol**

USES: **To treat moderate to severe pain**

FDA PREGNANCY CATEGORY: **C**

VIRTUALLY NO RISK	SLIGHT RISK	MODERATE RISK	STRONG RISK	EXTREME RISK

Currently, there are no reports regarding the use of Ultram in early human pregnancy. No birth defects have been reported with the use of this drug in animals. With a lack of proper data, the risk in the use of this drug during pregnancy cannot be assessed. Until further studies are available, this drug should be avoided during pregnancy.

BREAST-FEEDING: This drug is found in breast milk. The potential effects of exposure to this drug on a breast-feeding infant are not known. Nursing mothers taking this drug should use caution when breast-feeding.

BRAND NAME: **Urised**

GENERIC NAME: **Combination product containing methenamine, phenyl salicylate, methylene blue, benzoic acid, atropine, and hyoscyamine**

USES: **To treat urinary tract infections**

FDA PREGNANCY CATEGORY: **C**

VIRTUALLY NO RISK	SLIGHT RISK	MODERATE RISK	STRONG RISK	EXTREME RISK

Urised should be used with caution during pregnancy due to a lack of available data. There have been no animal or human studies to assess the possible occurrence of birth defects when using this drug. Hyoscyamine and atropine, two of the ingredients in this product, have been associated with a small percentage of birth defects. Until studies are conducted, Urised should be not used during pregnancy unless its benefits outweigh its potential risks to the fetus.

BREAST-FEEDING: It is not known whether the drug is found in breast milk. Caution should be used when breast-feeding.

BRAND NAME: **Valium**

GENERIC NAME: **diazepam**

USES: **To treat anxiety, muscle spasms, and seizures**

FDA PREGNANCY CATEGORY: **D**

VIRTUALLY NO RISK	SLIGHT RISK	MODERATE RISK	STRONG RISK	EXTREME RISK

Valium has been suspected of causing fetal abnormalities such as cleft lip and palate, slanted eyes, breathing problems, and hernia. This drug does cross the placenta and can cause "floppy infant syndrome." Floppy infant syndrome occurs at birth and its symptoms include tiredness and sucking difficulties. When a mother takes high doses during pregnancy, her baby can suffer withdrawal effects upon delivery, which include shakiness, diarrhea, vomiting, irritability, and slow growth. With these possible effects in mind, it is not advised to take Valium during pregnancy.

BREAST-FEEDING: This drug is found in breast milk. The potential effects of exposure to this drug on a breast-feeding infant are not known. Nursing mothers taking this drug should use extreme caution when breast-feeding.

BRAND NAME: **Valtrex**

GENERIC NAME: **valacyclovir**

USES: **To treat shingles and genital herpes**

FDA PREGNANCY CATEGORY: **B**

VIRTUALLY NO RISK	SLIGHT RISK	MODERATE RISK	STRONG RISK	EXTREME RISK

Valtrex is used to treat viruses that cause herpes, chicken pox, and shingles. It is converted to Zovirax by the body after it is taken. In several studies, Valtrex was found to have no adverse effects on the fetus; however, several reports of malformations have occurred with the use of Zovirax in pregnancy, including neural tube defects, cleft palate, and limb deformities. Miscarriage has also been reported. A definite relationship between the drug and these birth defects could not be proven, but the defects could have resulted from the mother's disease or exposure to other drugs. Valtrex should be used with caution during pregnancy.

BREAST-FEEDING: This drug is found in breast milk. The potential effects of exposure to this drug on a breast-feeding infant are not known. Nursing mothers taking this drug should use caution when breast-feeding.

BRAND NAME: **Vancenase AQ DS**
GENERIC NAME: **beclomethasone dipropionate**
USES: **To treat nasal allergies, nasal polyps, and nasal inflammation**
FDA PREGNANCY CATEGORY: **C**

VIRTUALLY NO RISK	SLIGHT RISK	MODERATE RISK	STRONG RISK	EXTREME RISK

Vancenase is a steroid that is inhaled through the nose and used in the treatment of nasal allergies and polyps. Like other steroids, beclamethasone has been shown to cause birth defects when given to mice and rabbits. No studies have been conducted in pregnant women to look at the effects of Vancenase AQ on the fetus. Due to the lack of safety data, Vancenase AQ is not recommended for use during pregnancy unless its potential benefits outweigh its potential risks to the fetus.

BREAST-FEEDING: This drug is found in breast milk. The potential effects of exposure to this drug on a breast-feeding infant are not known. Nursing mothers taking this drug should use some caution when breast-feeding.

BRAND NAME: **Vantin**

GENERIC NAME: **cefpodoxime**

USES: **To treat bacterial infections**

FDA PREGNANCY CATEGORY: **B**

VIRTUALLY NO RISK	SLIGHT RISK	MODERATE RISK	STRONG RISK	EXTREME RISK

Vantin is an antibiotic used to treat bacterial infections. It is generally considered safe for use during pregnancy. In rats given doses up to two times the recommended human dose, no adverse effects on the fetus were reported. No studies are available on the use of Vantin in human pregnancy.

BREAST-FEEDING: This drug is found in breast milk. The potential effects of exposure to this drug on a breast-feeding infant are not known. Nursing mothers taking this drug should use caution when breast-feeding.

BRAND NAME: **Vasotec**

GENERIC NAME: **enalapril**

USES: **To treat high blood pressure and heart failure**

FDA PREGNANCY CATEGORY: **D**

VIRTUALLY NO RISK	SLIGHT RISK	MODERATE RISK	STRONG RISK	EXTREME RISK

Vasotec should be used with extreme caution during pregnancy. In the second and third trimesters of pregnancy, this drug has been shown to cause severe birth defects and possible death of the fetus. During the first trimester of pregnancy, its safety is only slightly better. Therefore, this drug should not be used at all during pregnancy unless potential benefits strongly outweigh the very serious risks to the fetus.

BREAST-FEEDING: This drug is found in breast milk. The potential effects of exposure to this drug on a breast-feeding infant are not known. Nursing mothers taking this drug should use caution when breast-feeding.

BRAND NAME: **Veetids**

GENERIC NAME: **penicillin V potassium**

USES: **To treat bacterial infections**

FDA PREGNANCY CATEGORY: **B**

VIRTUALLY NO RISK	SLIGHT RISK	MODERATE RISK	STRONG RISK	EXTREME RISK

Penicillin is an antibiotic used to treat various bacterial infections. No conclusive reports on the use of penicillin in pregnancy have shown that the drug causes birth defects. Penicillin is generally considered fairly safe to use during pregnancy.

BREAST-FEEDING: It is not known whether the drug is found in breast milk. As with all drugs, some caution should be used when breast-feeding.

BRAND NAME: **Ventolin**

GENERIC NAME: **albuterol**

Same as **Proventil;** see entry for **Proventil**

BRAND NAME: **Verelan**

GENERIC NAME: **verapamil**

Same as **Calan;** see entry for **Calan**

BRAND NAME: **Vicodin**

GENERIC NAME: **Combination product containing acetaminophen and hydrocodone**

USES: **To alleviate moderate to severe pain**

FDA PREGNANCY CATEGORY: **C**

VIRTUALLY NO RISK	SLIGHT RISK	MODERATE RISK	STRONG RISK	EXTREME RISK

The acetaminophen component of this drug is safe to use during all stages of pregnancy. The drug should only be used for short periods of time, because long-term use can cause problems in the infant, such as anemia or a low red blood cell count. However, because of the hydrocodone component some caution is needed. Some birth defects have been found with the use of this drug in hamsters. One study looked at first-trimester exposure and found no evidence of birth defects. The hydrocodone component of this drug can cause withdrawal in infants if mothers use high doses. If Vicodin is used for prolonged periods or in high doses, this drug becomes more risky. Vicodin should be used with extreme caution during pregnancy.

BREAST-FEEDING: This drug is found in breast milk. The potential effects of exposure to this drug on a breast-feeding infant are not known. Nursing mothers taking this drug should use extreme caution when breast-feeding.

BRAND NAME: **Voltaren**
GENERIC NAME: **diclofenac sodium**
USES: **For relief of arthritis pain, menstrual pain, and other pain**
FDA PREGNANCY CATEGORY: **B**

VIRTUALLY NO RISK	SLIGHT RISK	MODERATE RISK	STRONG RISK	EXTREME RISK

When this drug is used in high doses during pregnancy, reported adverse effects in the fetus have been minimal. These effects included decreased fetal growth and lengthened delivery. In mice, cleft palate was noted. Also, this agent should be avoided in those trying to conceive because this drug can block implantation of the fertilized egg. When used near delivery or in the third trimester, this drug is classified as "more risky" because of the possible increase in blood pressure in the lungs of the fetus. Voltaren has also been shown to prolong pregnancies and slow down labor. This drug should be used with caution.

BREAST-FEEDING: This drug is found in breast milk. The potential effects of exposure to this drug on a breast-feeding infant are not known. Nursing mothers taking this drug should use caution when breast-feeding.

BRAND NAME: **Wellbutrin SR**
GENERIC NAME: **bupropion**
USES: **To treat depression**
FDA PREGNANCY CATEGORY: **B**

VIRTUALLY NO RISK	SLIGHT RISK	MODERATE RISK	STRONG RISK	EXTREME RISK

Adequate studies have not been performed on the use of this drug during pregnancy. In rats and rabbits receiving high doses of this drug, no harm to the fetus was observed. With minimal data available on this drug, caution should be advised and the drug should be used only if its benefits outweigh its risks.

BREAST-FEEDING: This drug is found in breast milk. The potential effects of exposure to this drug on a breast-feeding infant are not known. Nursing mothers taking this drug should use caution when breast-feeding.

BRAND NAME: **Xanax**
GENERIC NAME: **alprazolam**
Similar to **Valium;** see entry for **Valium**

BRAND NAME: **Zantac**

GENERIC NAME: **ranitidine**

USES: **To treat active stomach ulcers, active duodenal ulcers (ulcers of the upper part of the small intestine, also called peptic ulcers), maintenance of healed duodenal ulcers, and the treatment of gastroesophageal reflux disease (GERD)**

FDA PREGNANCY CATEGORY: **B**

VIRTUALLY NO RISK	SLIGHT RISK	MODERATE RISK	STRONG RISK	EXTREME RISK
▓	▓			

No problems have been associated with the use of this drug during pregnancy. In rats and rabbits, no birth defects were found. When used prior to delivery, no problems were noted in the newborn. Zantac is fairly safe to use during pregnancy under the supervision of a physician.

BREAST-FEEDING: This drug is found in breast milk. The potential effects of exposure to this drug on a breast-feeding infant are not known. Nursing mothers taking this drug should use some caution when breast-feeding.

BRAND NAME: **Zenate**

GENERIC NAME: **prenatal multivitamin**

Similar to **Natalins Rx;** see entry for **Natalins Rx**

BRAND NAME: **Zestoretic**

GENERIC NAME: **Combination product containing lisinopril and hydrochlorothiazide**

USES: **To treat high blood pressure and heart failure**

FDA PREGNANCY CATEGORY: **D**

VIRTUALLY NO RISK	SLIGHT RISK	MODERATE RISK	STRONG RISK	EXTREME RISK
▓	▓	▓	▓	

Zestoretic is a product that contains twp ingredients—lisinopril and hydrochlorothiazide. Lisinopril should be used with extreme caution during pregnancy. In the second and third trimesters, it has been shown to cause severe birth defects and possible death of the fetus. During the first trimester, its safety is only slightly better. Hydrochlorothiazide is also not recommended for use during pregnancy. Use of hydrochlorothiazide during the first trimester has been linked to birth defects. Use in the second and third trimesters has been linked to slow heart rate, low blood sugar, low sodium and potassium, and death in the fetus. Zestoretic should not be used at any time during pregnancy.

BREAST-FEEDING: This drug is found in breast milk. The potential effects of exposure to this drug on a breast-feeding infant are not known. Nursing mothers taking this drug should use caution when breast-feeding.

BRAND NAME: **Zestril**
GENERIC NAME: **lisinopril**
Similar to **Accupril;** see entry for **Accupril**

BRAND NAME: **Ziac**
GENERIC NAME: **Combination product containing bisoprolol and hydrochlorothiazide**
USES: **To treat high blood pressure**
FDA PREGNANCY CATEGORY: **D**

VIRTUALLY NO RISK	SLIGHT RISK	MODERATE RISK	STRONG RISK	EXTREME RISK

Ziac is a drug that contains two ingredients—bisoprolol and hydrochlorothiazide. It is not recommended for use during pregnancy. Bisoprolol has not been shown to cause any birth defects when studied in rats and rabbits; however, slowed growth and decreased weight of the fetus has been reported when the drug is taken during the second and third trimesters. Hydrochlorothiazide is also not recommended for use during pregnancy. Use of hydrochlorothiazide during the first trimester has been linked to birth defects. Use in the second and third trimesters has been linked to slow heart rate, low blood sugar, low sodium and potassium, and death in the fetus. Ziac should not be used at any time during pregnancy.

BREAST-FEEDING: This drug is found in breast milk. The potential effects of exposure to this drug on a breast-feeding infant are not known. Nursing mothers taking this drug should use caution when breast-feeding.

BRAND NAME: **Zithromax**
GENERIC NAME: **azithromycin**
USES: **To treat bacterial infections**
FDA PREGNANCY CATEGORY: **B**

VIRTUALLY NO RISK	SLIGHT RISK	MODERATE RISK	STRONG RISK	EXTREME RISK

Zithromax, a derivative of erythromycin, has been studied in animals at doses well above 600mg. These high doses, which would be toxic in humans, showed no impairment of fertility or harm to the fetus. Only two small studies have been conducted in pregnant women who needed Zithromax for treatment of chlamydia, and results from these pregnancies were not reported. Zithromax should be used with some caution during pregnancy until more research and clinical experience in pregnant women is available.

BREAST-FEEDING: This drug is found in breast milk. The potential effects of exposure to this drug on a breast-feeding infant are not known. Nursing mothers taking this drug should use caution when breast-feeding.

BRAND NAME: **Zocor**

GENERIC NAME: **simvastatin**

Very similar to **Mevacor;** see entry for **Mevacor**

BRAND NAME: **Zoloft**

GENERIC NAME: **sertraline**

USES: **To treat depression and obsessive-compulsive disorder**

FDA PREGNANCY CATEGORY: **B**

VIRTUALLY NO RISK	SLIGHT RISK	MODERATE RISK	STRONG RISK	EXTREME RISK

Limited studies have been done regarding the use of Zoloft during pregnancy. When this drug was taken during pregnancy, there was an increased risk of birth defects noted. In other drugs in the selective serotonin reuptake inhibitors (SSRIs) family, some minor malformations were identified, including heart problems. When taken during the third trimester, there is an increased risk of decreased birth weight and complications with fetal breathing. Prozac, another SSRI, apparently does not affect the development of the children who were exposed to this drug during pregnancy, whereas with Zoloft the same conclusion cannot be made without further data. With the lack of clinical evidence and experience with Zoloft available during pregnancy, Prozac should be chosen over Zoloft if there is a need to treat depression.

BREAST-FEEDING: This drug is found in breast milk. The potential effects of exposure to this drug on a breast-feeding infant are not known. Nursing mothers taking this drug should use caution when breast-feeding.

BRAND NAME: **Zovirax**

GENERIC NAME: **acyclovir**

USES: **To treat genital herpes, shingles, chicken pox, and herpes cold sores**

FDA PREGNANCY CATEGORY: **C**

VIRTUALLY NO RISK	SLIGHT RISK	MODERATE RISK	STRONG RISK	EXTREME RISK
▨	▨	▨		

Zovirax is used to treat many types of infections caused by viruses. The use of Zovirax during pregnancy is not recommended; however, the drug has been used to treat the herpes simplex virus in the mother. Several reports of malformations have occurred with the use of Zovirax during pregnancy, and they include neural tube defects, cleft palate, and limb deformities. Miscarriage has also been reported. A definite relationship between the drug and these birth defects could not be proven, but the defects could have resulted from the mother's disease or use of other drugs. Zovirax is not recommended for use during pregnancy unless its benefits strongly outweigh its risks to the fetus.

BREAST-FEEDING: This drug is found in breast milk. The American Academy of Pediatrics considers this drug to be compatible with breast-feeding. As with all drugs, some caution should still be used.

BRAND NAME: **Zyban**

GENERIC NAME: **bupropion**

Similar to **Wellbutrin SR;** see entry for **Wellbutrin SR**

BRAND NAME: **Zyflo**

GENERIC NAME: **zileuton**

USES: **To treat asthma and other breathing disorders**

FDA PREGNANCY CATEGORY: **C**

VIRTUALLY NO RISK	SLIGHT RISK	MODERATE RISK	STRONG RISK	EXTREME RISK

Zyflo is an oral drug used to prevent and treat asthma. In rats given doses higher than is suggested for human use, reduced fetal weight and changes in the fetal skeleton were observed. In rats, Zyflo has been found to cross the placenta. No adequate studies have been done examining the use of Zyflo and its effects in pregnant women. Due to the lack of safety data, Zyflo is not recommended for use during pregnancy unless its benefits strongly outweigh its potential risk to the fetus.

BREAST-FEEDING: It is not known whether the drug is found in breast milk. Caution should be used when breast-feeding.

BRAND NAME: **Zyprexa**

GENERIC NAME: **olanzapine**

USES: **To treat psychosis**

FDA PREGNANCY CATEGORY: **C**

VIRTUALLY NO RISK	SLIGHT RISK	MODERATE RISK	STRONG RISK	EXTREME RISK

Adequate studies regarding the use of this drug during pregnancy do not exist. In rats and rabbits, pregnancy was prolonged and miscarriages occurred, but no birth defects were noted. Seven human pregnancies were observed during which this drug was used. Miscarriage and heart problems in the fetuses occurred in some of women studied. This drug should be avoided unless its benefits to the patient clearly outweigh its risk to the fetus.

BREAST-FEEDING: This drug is found in breast milk and may be harmful to a breast-feeding infant. This drug should not be taken by nursing mothers.

BRAND NAME: **Zyrtec**

GENERIC NAME: **cetirizine**

USES: **To treat allergies**

FDA PREGNANCY CATEGORY: **B**

VIRTUALLY NO RISK	SLIGHT RISK	MODERATE RISK	STRONG RISK	EXTREME RISK

Zyrtec is an oral drug used in the treatment of allergies and itching. There are no studies of Zyrtec use by pregnant women. However, in mice, rats, and rabbits given doses above the maximum recommended human dose, no adverse effects to the fetus were reported. Due to the lack of studies involving Zyrtec and human pregnancy, it should be used with some caution.

BREAST-FEEDING: This drug is found in breast milk. The potential effects of exposure to this drug on a breast-feeding infant are not known. Nursing mothers taking this drug should use caution when breast-feeding.

CHAPTER 3

Over-the-Counter Products and Pregnancy

Almost none of the over-the-counter drugs have been tested in pregnant women to determine their potential effects on the fetus. This is not surprising since it would be unethical to just test these products on unknowing patients. Many of these products have been tested on animals. Scientists try to draw conclusions about humans based on the findings in animals. Human fetal development is inherently different from animal development, so precise conclusions regarding the effect of a drug on humans based on animal models is not always completely accurate, but it is often all that is available. Some of our knowledge of a drug's effect on the fetus comes from past experience. Documented case reports on the effects of a drug on the fetus provide health care professionals with some useful information, but understanding the true effect on the fetus is not an exact science. Many consumers view over-the-counter medications as safer than prescription ones. When used during pregnancy, this is not always the case. Even though these drugs do not require a prescription, they are still potent pharmacological agents. Some over-the-counter medications can cause potentially serious birth defects. This chapter provides some detailed information regarding the potential risk to the fetus from the most popular over-the-counter medications. However before using any over-the-counter product, always consult your doctor and/or pharmacist first!

BRAND NAME: **Actifed**

GENERIC NAME: **Combination product containing pseudoephedrine and triprolidine**

USES: **To treat the common cold, allergies, and congestion**

FDA PREGNANCY CATEGORY: **C**

VIRTUALLY NO RISK	SLIGHT RISK	MODERATE RISK	STRONG RISK	EXTREME RISK

Actifed is a drug used to relieve various symptoms associated with allergic disorders and common colds. Actifed contains two active ingredients—pseudoephedrine and triprolidine. Pseudoephedrine, and other drugs in this same category, has been shown to cause birth defects in animals. Exposure to pseudoephedrine during the first trimester has shown a significantly increased risk of fetal malformations. Many physicians suggest avoiding pseudoephedrine during the first trimester of pregnancy and using some caution during the second and third trimesters. The second ingredient, triprolidine, is an antihistamine used to treat various allergic symptoms. Studies conducted in humans on the use of triprolidine during pregnancy have not shown a definitive causal relationship between the drug and birth defects, but more research is needed. Actifed is not recommended for use during pregnancy unless its benefits outweigh its potential risks to the fetus.

BREAST-FEEDING: This drug is found in breast milk. The American Academy of Pediatrics considers this drug to be compatible with breast-feeding. As with all drugs, some caution should still be used.

BRAND NAME: **Advil**

GENERIC NAME: **ibuprofen**

USES: **To treat minor aches and pains of arthritis and reduce fever**

FDA PREGNANCY CATEGORY: **C**

VIRTUALLY NO RISK	SLIGHT RISK	MODERATE RISK	STRONG RISK	EXTREME RISK

Advil is a nonsteroidal anti-inflammatory drug (NSAID) used to treat pain and inflammation. No published studies regarding the use of Advil in humans exist; however, several case reports of its use during pregnancy have shown a small percentage of birth defects, including cardiovascular disorders, oral clefts, and spina bifida. Advil should absolutely not be taken during the third trimester because of the possibility of high blood pressure in the lungs of the fetus. Inhibition of labor and longer pregnancies has also been associated with the use of Advil during the third trimester. Women who are trying to become pregnant should also avoid the use of Advil because of animal studies that indicate it may prevent a fertilized egg from implanting in the uterus properly. The use of Advil during pregnancy should only be considered if its benefits outweigh its potential risks to the fetus.

BREAST-FEEDING: This drug is found in breast milk. The American Academy of Pediatrics considers this drug to be compatible with breast-feeding. As with all drugs, some caution should still be used.

BRAND NAME: **Afrin**
GENERIC NAME: **oxymetalozine**
USES: **Topical nasal decongestant**
FDA PREGNANCY CATEGORY: **C**

VIRTUALLY NO RISK	SLIGHT RISK	MODERATE RISK	STRONG RISK	EXTREME RISK

Afrin is a blood vessel constrictor that is used as a nasal decongestant. The use of Afrin has not been associated with any birth defects; however, studies have not included enough women to rule out the possibility of fetal abnormalities. The use of Afrin could potentially cause a decrease in the delivery of blood to the fetus, thus decreasing oxygen delivery to the fetus, which could result in a slowed fetal heart rate. Afrin should be used with caution during pregnancy.

BREAST-FEEDING: It is not known whether the drug is found in breast milk. Caution should be used when breast-feeding.

BRAND NAME: **Alka-Seltzer**

GENERIC NAME: **Combination product containing sodium bicarbonate and potassium bicarbonate**

USES: **To relieve acid indigestion and heartburn**

FDA PREGNANCY CATEGORY: **C**

VIRTUALLY NO RISK	SLIGHT RISK	MODERATE RISK	STRONG RISK	EXTREME RISK
▨	▨	▨		

Alka-Seltzer is a drug that is dissolved in water and used to treat the various symptoms of upset stomach and colds or allergies. The bicarbonate contained in Alka-Seltzer should be avoided during pregnancy due to its potential to induce sodium and water retention, which could eventually lead to high blood pressure. Some Alka-Seltzer products also contain aspirin. Aspirin is potentially the most common and most dangerous drug taken during pregnancy. In general, long-term use should be avoided because it can cause an increase in the risk of bleeding in the fetus at any time. High doses (650mg to 1,000mg) should be avoided, especially during the last three months of pregnancy. Lower doses should also be avoided in the last trimester because they have been associated with heart problems in the fetus. Alka-Seltzer is not recommended for use during pregnancy unless its benefits outweigh its potential risks to the fetus.

BREAST-FEEDING: It is not known whether the drug is found in breast milk. Caution should be used when breast-feeding.

BRAND NAME: **Anusol ointment**

GENERIC NAME: **Combination product containing pramoxine and zinc oxide**

USES: **To treat hemorrhoids**

FDA PREGNANCY CATEGORY: **C**

VIRTUALLY NO RISK	SLIGHT RISK	MODERATE RISK	STRONG RISK	EXTREME RISK
▨	▨	▨		

Anusol is a topical ointment used for the treatment of hemorrhoids. According to the manufacturer, there have been no studies conducted to determine its effects on the fetus if used during pregnancy; therefore, Anusol should be used with caution during pregnancy.

BREAST-FEEDING: This drug is not found in breast milk. Women may breast-feed while using this preparation.

BRAND NAME: **Aspirin**

GENERIC NAME: **aspirin**

See entry for **Bayer Aspirin**

BRAND NAME: **Axid AR**

GENERIC NAME: **nizatidine**

USES: **For the prevention of heartburn, acid indigestion, and sour stomach**

FDA PREGNANCY CATEGORY: **B**

VIRTUALLY NO RISK	SLIGHT RISK	MODERATE RISK	STRONG RISK	EXTREME RISK
▨	▨			

Axid is a drug used to block the effects of excess acid secretion in the stomach. Axid crosses the placenta. When given to pregnant rats and rabbits, no birth defects were reported in doses up to 1,500mg per kilogram of body weight. However, at the highest doses, abortions occurred in rabbits. Other birth defects, including spina bifida and an enlarged heart, were identified at lower doses in rabbits. With this information in mind, Axid should be used with some caution during pregnancy.

BREAST-FEEDING: This drug is found in breast milk. The potential effects of exposure to this drug on a breast-feeding infant are not known. Nursing mothers taking this drug should use caution when breast-feeding.

BRAND NAME: **Bayer Aspirin**

GENERIC NAME: **aspirin**

USES: **To treat headache, pain, fever, muscular aches and pains, and minor arthritis pain**

FDA PREGNANCY CATEGORY: **C**

VIRTUALLY NO RISK	SLIGHT RISK	MODERATE RISK	STRONG RISK	EXTREME RISK

Aspirin is probably the most frequently taken drug during pregnancy and it can be dangerous. In general, long-term use of aspirin should be avoided at any time during pregnancy. Aspirin can increase the risk of significant bleeding in the fetus anytime during pregnancy. Also, high doses (650mg to 1,000mg) should be avoided as well, especially during the last trimester of pregnancy. During the last trimester, doses as low as two regular-strength aspirin tablets may cause heart abnormalities in the fetus. Aspirin may also increase delivery and labor time. Aspirin absolutely should never be used during the last three months of pregnancy. The only exception is when low doses may be beneficial, such as in pregnancy-induced high blood pressure or preeclampsia. Acetaminophen (Tylenol®) is the best and safest choice for pain relief during pregnancy.

BREAST-FEEDING: This drug is found in breast milk and may be harmful to a breast-feeding infant. This drug should not be taken by nursing mothers.

BRAND NAME: **Benadryl**

GENERIC NAME: **diphenhydramine**

USES: **To treat upper respiratory allergies, and sneezing due to the common cold**

FDA PREGNANCY CATEGORY: **B**

VIRTUALLY NO RISK	SLIGHT RISK	MODERATE RISK	STRONG RISK	EXTREME RISK

Benadryl is an antihistamine used to treat allergies and insomnia. Rats and rabbits who received doses up to 5 times the normal human dose showed no fetal harm. However, some studies have reported birth defects, including hernias, cardiovascular disorders, urinary abnormalities, and eye and ear defects. Benadryl has also been shown to cause some uterine contractions. No direct relationship between the use of Benadryl and these birth defects has been proven. Abnormalities could have been a result of the mother's disease and/or other drug use. The use of antihistamines during the last two weeks of pregnancy has been associated with retrolental fibroplasia, a fibrous tissue deposit behind the lens of the eye, causing blindness in some prematurely born infants. Benadryl should never be used during the last two weeks of pregnancy. At other times, Benadryl should be used with caution during pregnancy.

BREAST-FEEDING: This drug is found in breast milk and may be harmful to a breast-feeding infant. This drug should not be taken by nursing mothers.

BRAND NAME: **Bonine**

GENERIC NAME: **meclizine**

USES: **To treat nausea, vomiting, and dizziness associated with motion sickness**

FDA PREGNANCY CATEGORY: **C**

VIRTUALLY NO RISK	SLIGHT RISK	MODERATE RISK	STRONG RISK	EXTREME RISK

Bonine is an antihistamine used to prevent and treat motion sickness. Bonine has been shown to cause birth defects in animals. In one human study, reported birth defects following exposure to Bonine included respiratory defects, hernias, and defects in the eyes and ears. The actual risk associated with Bonine use during pregnancy is not known. The use of antihistamines during the last two weeks of pregnancy has been associated with retrolental fibroplasia, a fibrous tissue deposit behind the lens of the eye, causing blindness in some prematurely born infants. Bonine should never be used during the last two weeks of pregnancy. Bonine is not recommended for use during pregnancy at all unless its benefits outweigh its potential risks to the fetus.

BREAST-FEEDING: This drug is found in breast milk. The potential effects of exposure to this drug on a breast-feeding infant are not known. Nursing mothers taking this drug should use caution when breast-feeding.

BRAND NAME: **Bufferin**
GENERIC NAME: **aspirin**
See entry for **Bayer Aspirin**

BRAND NAME: **Caladryl**
GENERIC NAME: **Combination product containing calamine and diphenhydramine**
USES: **To provide relief of itching due to mild poison ivy, insect bites, or other minor skin irritations**
FDA PREGNANCY CATEGORY: **C**

VIRTUALLY NO RISK	SLIGHT RISK	MODERATE RISK	STRONG RISK	EXTREME RISK

Caladryl is a topical product applied to the skin for the relief of symptoms associated with poison ivy. Caladryl contains two active ingredients—calamine and diphenhydramine. The use of diphenhydramine in rats and rabbits receiving oral doses up to 5 times the normal human dose showed no fetal harm. The use of antihistamines during the last two weeks of pregnancy has been associated with retrolental fibroplasia, a fibrous tissue deposit behind the lens of the eye, causing blindness in some prematurely born infants. Calamine has not been extensively studied in pregnant women and its potential effects on a developing fetus are unknown. Caladryl should never be used during the last two weeks of pregnancy and should be used with caution at other times during pregnancy.

BREAST-FEEDING: This drug is found in breast milk. The potential effects of exposure to this drug on a breast-feeding infant are not known. Nursing mothers taking this drug should use caution when breast-feeding.

BRAND NAME: **Caltrate**
GENERIC NAME: **calcium carbonate**
USES: **Vitamin supplement**
FDA PREGNANCY CATEGORY: **B**

VIRTUALLY NO RISK	SLIGHT RISK	MODERATE RISK	STRONG RISK	EXTREME RISK

Calcium is a mineral needed for the proper maintenance of bones, teeth, and other vital body functions. A pregnant woman has an increased requirement for calcium as her body provides nutrition to the developing fetus. Calcium carbonate is one supplement that may be taken to increase the daily calcium intake. Food sources rich in calcium include milk, cheeses, and other dairy products; they should also be consumed in larger amounts during pregnancy. Consultation with a physician is recommended to determine the proper amount of vitamin/mineral supplementation required during pregnancy.

BREAST-FEEDING: This product is not found in breast milk. Women may breast-feed while taking this drug.

BRAND NAME: **Chloraseptic**

GENERIC NAME: **phenol**

USES: **To treat minor sore throat pain**

FDA PREGNANCY CATEGORY: **C**

VIRTUALLY NO RISK	SLIGHT RISK	MODERATE RISK	STRONG RISK	EXTREME RISK

Chloraseptic is a drug that is usually sprayed into the throat for the relief of pain and irritation. According to the manufacturer, no clinical studies have been conducted to determine the effects on the fetus of Chloraseptic use during pregnancy. Chloraseptic is a product that is applied topically, therefore absorption into the bloodstream is less concentrated than if an oral dose of the drug was given. Due to the lack of information regarding Chloraseptic use during pregnancy, some caution should be taken with this product.

BREAST-FEEDING: This drug is found in breast milk. The potential effects of exposure to this drug on a breast-feeding infant are not known. Nursing mothers using this drug should use some caution when breast-feeding.

BRAND NAME: **Chlor-Trimeton**

GENERIC NAME: **chlorpheniramine**

USES: **To provide relief of seasonal allergies**

FDA PREGNANCY CATEGORY: **C**

VIRTUALLY NO RISK	SLIGHT RISK	MODERATE RISK	STRONG RISK	EXTREME RISK

Chlor-Trimeton is an antihistamine used to treat the symptoms of various allergic disorders. Birth defects caused by the use of Chlor-Trimeton during pregnancy have not been proven; however, some malformations have been reported following exposure during pregnancy. Some of the malformations included gastrointestinal disorders, hernias, hip dislocations, and eye and ear defects. The use of antihistamines during the last

two weeks of pregnancy has been associated with retrolental fibroplasia, a fibrous tissue deposit behind the lens of the eye, causing blindness in some prematurely born infants. Chlor-Trimeton should never be
used during the last two weeks of pregnancy. Chlor-Trimeton is not recommended for use during pregnancy unless its benefits outweigh its potential risks to the fetus.

BREAST-FEEDING: It is not known whether the drug is found in breast milk.
Caution should be used when breast-feeding.

BRAND NAME: **Citrucel**
GENERIC NAME: **methylcellulose**
USES: **As a bulk-forming fiber laxative**
FDA PREGNANCY CATEGORY: **B**

VIRTUALLY NO RISK	SLIGHT RISK	MODERATE RISK	STRONG RISK	EXTREME RISK

Citrucel is a bulk-forming laxative used to treat constipation. It is generally considered safe for use during pregnancy. Increasing dietary fiber
is the most common recommendation for treating constipation during
pregnancy. The drug may cause diarrhea in a small number of patients.
If prolonged diarrhea occurs, the potential for imbalances in electrolytes
(sodium, potassium, etc.) may occur as well as a loss of important nutrients vital for fetal growth and development. Citrucel should be used
with some caution during pregnancy. To treat constipation, increasing
dietary fiber intake should be attempted before any drug therapy is ini-
tiated.

BREAST-FEEDING: Citrucel is not found in breast milk. Women may breast-
feed while taking it.

BRAND NAME: **Clearasil**

GENERIC NAME: **salicyclic acid (topical)**

USES: **To treat acne**

FDA PREGNANCY CATEGORY: **C**

VIRTUALLY NO RISK	SLIGHT RISK	MODERATE RISK	STRONG RISK	EXTREME RISK

Clearasil is a topical product used for the treatment of acne. Although it is applied externally to the skin, some absorption into the bloodstream may occur. The active ingredient in Clearasil, salicylic acid, is a derivative of aspirin. Aspirin is probably the most frequently taken drug during pregnancy and it can be dangerous. In general, long-term use of aspirin should be avoided at any time during pregnancy. Aspirin can increase the risk of significant bleeding in the fetus anytime during pregnancy. Also, high doses (650mg to 1,000mg) should be avoided as well, especially during the last trimester of pregnancy. During the last trimester, doses as low as two regular-strength aspirin tablets may cause heart abnormalities in the fetus. Aspirin may also increase delivery and labor time. Aspirin should absolutely never be used during the last three months of pregnancy. Regular face washing with antibacterial soap and water is preferable to combat acne during pregnancy.

BREAST-FEEDING: This drug is found in breast milk. The potential effects of exposure to this drug on a breast-feeding infant are not known. Nursing mothers taking this drug should use caution when breast-feeding.

BRAND NAME: **Colace**

GENERIC NAME: **docusate**

USES: **As a stool softener**

FDA PREGNANCY CATEGORY: **C**

VIRTUALLY NO RISK	SLIGHT RISK	MODERATE RISK	STRONG RISK	EXTREME RISK

Colace, a common component of many laxatives, is used to treat constipation. The use of Colace during pregnancy has not been positively associated with birth defects; however, a very small percentage of malformations were reported following exposure to Colace during the first trimester. In one case, the use of Colace throughout pregnancy was suspected of causing a decreased amount of magnesium in the fetus. Colace should be used during pregnancy only under the supervision of a doctor.

BREAST-FEEDING: It is not known whether the drug is found in breast milk. Caution should be used when breast-feeding.

BRAND NAME: **Contac 12-hour**

GENERIC NAME: **Combination product containing pseudoephedrine and chlorpheniramine**

USES: **To treat nasal congestion due to the common cold or seasonal allergies**

FDA PREGNANCY CATEGORY: **C**

VIRTUALLY NO RISK	SLIGHT RISK	MODERATE RISK	STRONG RISK	EXTREME RISK

Contac is used to relieve nasal stuffiness associated with allergies and colds. Contac contains two active ingredients—pseudoephedrine and chlorpheniramine. Pseudoephedrine is used to relieve congestion associated with allergies and colds. It has been shown to cause birth defects in some animals. Exposure to pseudoephedrine during the first trimester has shown a significantly increased risk of fetal malformations. Many physicians suggest avoiding pseudoephedrine during the first trimester of pregnancy and to use some caution during the second and third trimesters. Birth defects caused by the use of chlorpheniramine during pregnancy have not been proven; however, some malformations have been reported following exposure during pregnancy. Some of the malformations included gastrointestinal disorders, hernias, hip dislocations,

and eye and ear defects. The use of antihistamines such as chlorpheniramine during the last two weeks of pregnancy has been associated
with retrolental fibroplasia, a fibrous tissue deposit behind the lens of
the eye, causing blindness in some prematurely born infants. Contac
should never be used during the last two weeks of pregnancy. At other
times during pregnancy, it should be used with caution.

BREAST-FEEDING: It is not known whether the drug is found in breast milk.
Caution should be used when breast-feeding.

BRAND NAME: **Correctol**
GENERIC NAME: **bisacodyl**
USES: **To treat constipation**
FDA PREGNANCY CATEGORY: **C**

VIRTUALLY NO RISK	SLIGHT RISK	MODERATE RISK	STRONG RISK	EXTREME RISK

Correctol is used to relieve constipation. Laxatives should be used very
cautiously in pregnancy because of the potential for causing diarrhea,
which depletes important electrolytes needed for proper growth and development of the fetus. Some of these electrolytes include sodium,
potassium, and magnesium. Correctol is a stimulant laxative and other
stimulant laxatives have been shown to induce premature labor. Correctol is not recommended for use during pregnancy unless its benefits
outweigh its potential risks to the fetus.

BREAST-FEEDING: It is not known whether the drug is found in breast milk.
Caution should be used when breast-feeding.

BRAND NAME: **Cortaid**

GENERIC NAME: **hydrocortisone**

USES: **To treat minor skin irritations and rashes**

FDA PREGNANCY CATEGORY: **C**

VIRTUALLY NO RISK	SLIGHT RISK	MODERATE RISK	STRONG RISK	EXTREME RISK

Cortaid is a topically applied steroid used for the treatment of skin irritation and rash. Even though the drug is applied externally to the skin, some of the drug is still absorbed into the bloodstream. Steroids are generally not considered safe for use during pregnancy because of adverse effects noted in both animals and humans. Exposure to hydrocortisone during the first trimester of pregnancy has resulted in birth defects, including cataracts, defects within the heart, clubfoot, undescended testes, and cleft lip. Cortaid is not recommended for use during pregnancy unless its benefits significantly outweigh its potential risks to the fetus.

BREAST-FEEDING: This drug is found in breast milk. The American Academy of Pediatrics considers this preparation to be compatible with breast-feeding. As with all drugs, some caution should still be used.

BRAND NAME: **Dimetapp**

GENERIC NAME: **Combination product containing pseudoephedrine and brompheniramine**

USES: **To treat the common cold or sinusitis**

FDA PREGNANCY CATEGORY: **C**

VIRTUALLY NO RISK	SLIGHT RISK	MODERATE RISK	STRONG RISK	EXTREME RISK

Dimetapp is a drug used to break up mucous and calm the coughing sensation. Dimetapp is a combination of two ingredients—pseudoephedrine and brompheniramine. Pseudoephedrine is used to relieve congestion associated with allergies and colds. It has been shown to cause birth defects in some animals. Exposure to pseudoephedrine during the first trimester has shown a significantly increased risk of fetal malformations. Many physicians suggest avoiding pseudoephedrine during the first trimester of pregnancy and to use some caution during the second and third trimesters. Brompheniramine is an antihistamine used to treat various symptoms of allergic disorders. In one study analyzing exposure to brompheniramine in 65 infants, a significant relationship between first-trimester drug use and fetal abnormalities was noted. The use of antihistamines during the last two weeks of pregnancy has been associated with retrolental fibroplasia, a fibrous tissue deposit behind the lens of the eye, causing blindness in some prematurely born infants. Dimetapp is not recommended for use during pregnancy unless its benefits outweigh its potential risks to the fetus.

BREAST-FEEDING: This drug is found in breast milk. The potential effects of exposure to this drug on a breast-feeding infant are not known. Nursing mothers taking this drug should use caution when breast-feeding.

BRAND NAME: **Doan's Pills**
GENERIC NAME: **magnesium salicylate**
USES: **For relief of minor backache**
FDA PREGNANCY CATEGORY: **C**

VIRTUALLY NO RISK	SLIGHT RISK	MODERATE RISK	STRONG RISK	EXTREME RISK

Doan's Pills are used to relieve general aches and pains, primarily back pains. The active ingredient in Doan's is magnesium salicylate. In general, salicylates, which are very similar to aspirin, should be avoided during pregnancy. Aspirin is probably the most frequently taken drug during pregnancy and it can be dangerous. In general, long-term use of aspirin should be avoided at any time during pregnancy. Aspirin can increase the risk of significant bleeding in the fetus anytime during pregnancy.

Also, high doses (650mg to 1,000mg) should be avoided as well, especially during the last trimester of pregnancy. During the last trimester, doses as low as two regular-strength aspirin tablets may cause heart abnormalities in the fetus. Aspirin may also increase delivery and labor time. Aspirin absolutely should never be used during the last three months of pregnancy. The only exception is when low doses may be beneficial, such as in pregnancy-induced high blood pressure or preeclampsia. Acetaminophen (Tylenol®) is the best and safest choice for pain relief during pregnancy.

BREAST-FEEDING: This drug is found in breast milk and may be harmful to a breast-feeding infant. This drug should not be taken by nursing mothers.

BRAND NAME: **Doxidan**
GENERIC NAME: **Combination product containing casanthranol and docusate**
USES: **To treat constipation**
FDA PREGNANCY CATEGORY: **C**

VIRTUALLY NO RISK	SLIGHT RISK	MODERATE RISK	STRONG RISK	EXTREME RISK

Doxidan is a drug used to treat constipation. Its two ingredients are casanthranol and docusate. An association between the use of casanthranol and birth defects has not been established; however, a small percentage of infants exposed to casanthranol during the first trimester displayed major birth defects. Some of these birth defects included cardiovascular defects, spina bifida, and limb abnormalities. The use of docusate during pregnancy has not been positively associated with birth defects; however, a very small percentage of malformations were reported following exposure to docusate during the first trimester. In one case, the use of docusate pregnancy was suspected of causing a decreased amount of magnesium in the fetus. Doxidan is not recommended for use during pregnancy unless its benefits outweigh its potential risks to the fetus.

BREAST-FEEDING: It is not known whether the drug is found in breast milk. Caution should be used when breast-feeding.

BRAND NAME: **Drixoral**

GENERIC NAME: **Combination product containing pseudoephedrine and dexbrompheniramine**

USES: **To treat nasal congestion due to the common cold and/or seasonal allergies**

FDA PREGNANCY CATEGORY: **C**

VIRTUALLY NO RISK	SLIGHT RISK	MODERATE RISK	STRONG RISK	EXTREME RISK
▓	▓	▓		

Drixoral is a drug used to alleviate the common signs and symptoms associated with a cold. Drixoral contains two active ingredients—pseudoephedrine and dexbrompheniramine. Pseudoephedrine, and other drugs in this category, has been shown to cause birth defects in animals. Exposure to pseudoephedrine during the first trimester has shown a significantly increased risk of fetal malformations. Many physicians suggest avoiding pseudoephedrine during the first trimester of pregnancy and using some caution during the second and third trimesters. Dexbrompheniramine is very similar to brompheniramine, an active ingredient in Dimetapp. Brompheniramine is an antihistamine used to treat various symptoms of allergic disorders. In one study analyzing exposure to brompheniramine in 65 infants, a significant relationship between first-trimester drug use and fetal abnormalities was noted. The use of antihistamines during the last two weeks of pregnancy has been associated with retrolental fibroplasia, a fibrous tissue deposit behind the lens of the eye, causing blindness in some prematurely born infants. Drixoral is not recommended for use during pregnancy unless its benefits outweigh its potential risks to the fetus.

BREAST-FEEDING: This drug is found in breast milk. The potential effects of exposure to this drug on a breast-feeding infant are not known. Nursing mothers taking this drug should use caution when breast-feeding.

BRAND NAME: **Dulcolax**
GENERIC NAME: **bisacodyl**
Same as **Correctol;** see entry for **Correctol**

BRAND NAME: **Ecotrin**
GENERIC NAME: **enteric-coated aspirin**
See entry for **Bayer Aspirin**

BRAND NAME: **Emetrol**
GENERIC NAME: **dextrose and fructose**
USES: **To treat nausea**
FDA PREGNANCY CATEGORY: **C**

VIRTUALLY NO RISK	SLIGHT RISK	MODERATE RISK	STRONG RISK	EXTREME RISK

Emetrol is used for the treatment of nausea and vomiting. According to the manufacturer, there have been no studies conducted to determine its effects on a developing fetus. Until more research is conducted, Emetrol should be used with caution during pregnancy.

BREAST-FEEDING: This drug is not found in breast milk. Women may breast-feed while taking this drug.

BRAND NAME: **Ex-Lax**

GENERIC NAME: **senna**

USES: **To treat constipation**

FDA PREGNANCY CATEGORY: **C**

VIRTUALLY NO RISK	SLIGHT RISK	MODERATE RISK	STRONG RISK	EXTREME RISK

Ex-Lax is used to treat constipation and contains a naturally occurring compound called senna. Ex-Lax is converted to an active drug by enzymes within the intestines. The use of Ex-Lax has shown no birth defects when studied in animals, and no reports of birth defects in humans have been established. The drug may cause diarrhea in a small number of patients. Diarrhea is something that must be monitored very closely during pregnancy. If prolonged diarrhea occurs, the potential for imbalances in electrolytes (sodium, potassium, etc.) may occur. The use of Ex-Lax is not recommended during pregnancy except under the care of a doctor.

BREAST-FEEDING: This drug is found in breast milk. The American Academy of Pediatrics considers this drug to be compatible with breast-feeding. As with all drugs, some caution should still be used.

BRAND NAME: **Excedrin Extra Strength and Excedrin Migraine**
GENERIC NAME: **Combination product containing acetaminophen, aspirin, and caffeine**
USES: **To treat headache, muscle aches, menstrual cramps, and minor arthritis pain**
FDA PREGNANCY CATEGORY: **C**

VIRTUALLY NO RISK	SLIGHT RISK	MODERATE RISK	STRONG RISK	EXTREME RISK

Excedrin is a combination product used to relieve various types of pain. Excedrin contains three active ingredients—acetaminophen, aspirin, and caffeine. Acetaminophen (Tylenol®) is generally considered safe for use during all trimesters of pregnancy for short-term pain relief and fever reduction. Unlike aspirin, acetaminophen does not interfere with platelet function and therefore does not cause a problem with bleeding when given near delivery. Aspirin is probably the most frequently taken drug during pregnancy and can be dangerous. In general, long-term use of aspirin should be avoided at any time during pregnancy. Aspirin can increase the risk of significant bleeding in the fetus anytime during pregnancy. Also, high doses (650mg to 1,000mg) should be avoided as well, especially during the last three months of pregnancy. During the last trimester of pregnancy, doses as low as two regular-strength aspirin tablets may cause heart abnormalities in the fetus. Aspirin may also increase delivery and labor time. Therefore, aspirin absolutely should never be used during the last three months of pregnancy. Acetaminophen (Tylenol®) alone is the best and safest choice for pain relief in women who are pregnant. High doses of caffeine may be responsible for miscarriage, difficulty in becoming pregnant, and infertility. Increased heart and breathing rates have been observed in the fetus of a mother who has been exposed to high amounts of caffeine. This product should not be considered for use during pregnancy unless its benefits strongly outweigh its potential risks to the fetus.

BREAST-FEEDING: This drug is found in breast milk and may be harmful to a breast-feeding infant. This drug should not be taken by nursing mothers.

BRAND NAME: **Femstat-3**
GENERIC NAME: **butoconazole**
USES: **To treat yeast infections**
FDA PREGNANCY CATEGORY: **C**

VIRTUALLY NO RISK	SLIGHT RISK	MODERATE RISK	STRONG RISK	EXTREME RISK

Femstat-3 is used in the treatment of vaginal fungal infections. This drug has been shown to cause birth defects in animals when administered in large oral doses. However, only 5.5 percent of a Femstat application is absorbed from the vagina into the bloodstream, which may lower the risk of birth defects. In an observational study conducted in Michigan, a small percentage of birth defects (including cardiovascular defects and spina bifida) were reported after human exposure during the first trimester. Use of the vaginal applicator could also potentially harm the uterus during pregnancy. Using Femstat-3 during pregnancy is not recommended unless its benefits outweigh its potential risks to the fetus.

BREAST-FEEDING: It is not known whether the drug is found in breast milk. Caution should be used when breast-feeding.

BRAND NAME: **Fleet Enema**
GENERIC NAME: **sodium biphosphate**
USES: **To treat constipation**
FDA PREGNANCY CATEGORY: **C**

VIRTUALLY NO RISK	SLIGHT RISK	MODERATE RISK	STRONG RISK	EXTREME RISK

Fleet Enema is used for the treatment of constipation. The active ingredient, sodium biphosphate, should be avoided during pregnancy because of its potential to induce sodium and water retention. This water retention has the potential to cause high blood pressure. The use of an enema could cause diarrhea, a condition that must be monitored very closely in pregnancy. If prolonged diarrhea occurs, imbalances in electrolytes (sodium, potassium, etc.) may occur, as well as loss of important nutrients vital for fetal growth and development. Fleet Enema is not recommended for use during pregnancy unless its benefits outweigh its potential risks to the fetus.

BREAST-FEEDING: This drug is not found in breast milk. Women may breast-feed while using this drug.

BRAND NAME: **Gas-X**
GENERIC NAME: **simethicone**
USES: **To relieve flatulence (gas)**
FDA PREGNANCY CATEGORY: **C**

VIRTUALLY NO RISK	SLIGHT RISK	MODERATE RISK	STRONG RISK	EXTREME RISK

Gas-X is used to relieve the pain and pressure associated with excess gas. No published reports are available that establish a positive relationship between Gas-X and birth defects. However, one case report did potentially establish a link between the drug and a cardiovascular birth defect. Gas-X should be used with caution during pregnancy.

BREAST-FEEDING: It is not known whether the drug is found in breast milk. Some caution should be used when breast-feeding.

BRAND NAME: **Gaviscon**
GENERIC NAME: **Combination product containing aluminum hydroxide, magnesium trisilicate, and alginic acid**
USES: **For relief of heartburn due to acid reflux**
FDA PREGNANCY CATEGORY: **C**

VIRTUALLY NO RISK	SLIGHT RISK	MODERATE RISK	STRONG RISK	EXTREME RISK

Gaviscon is used to treat the various symptoms associated with upset stomach and heartburn, both very common problems in pregnancy. Studies conducted in animals have shown no adverse effects when constant administration of antacids was performed. However, human studies are limited. All antacids have the potential to interfere with normal iron absorption, while aluminum-containing antacids have the potential to induce constipation. There have also been reports of muscle tendon problems in the fetuses of mothers who took high doses of antacids for long periods of time during pregnancy. No data is available to determine if alginic acid or magnesium trisilicate may cause harm to the fetus if taken during pregnancy. Gaviscon should be used with caution during pregnancy.

BREAST-FEEDING: It is not known whether the drug is found in breast milk. Some caution should be used when breast-feeding.

BRAND NAME: **Gyne-Lotrimin**
GENERIC NAME: **clotrimazole**
USES: **To treat vaginal yeast infections**
FDA PREGNANCY CATEGORY: **B**

VIRTUALLY NO RISK	SLIGHT RISK	MODERATE RISK	STRONG RISK	EXTREME RISK

Gyne-Lotrimin is used to treat various vaginal fungal infections. The use of Gyne-Lotrimin has not been proven to cause birth defects. However, a small percentage of birth defects in infants exposed to Gyne-Lotrimin during the first trimester were reported. Some of these defects included cardiovascular disorders, spina bifida, and disorders of the male reproductive organs. The use of a vaginal applicator may injure the uterus. Gyne-Lotrimin should be used with caution during pregnancy and only under the care of a physician.

BREAST-FEEDING: It is not known whether the drug is found in breast milk. Some caution should be used when breast-feeding.

BRAND NAME: **Imodium AD**

GENERIC NAME: **loperamide**

USES: **To treat diarrhea**

FDA PREGNANCY CATEGORY: **B**

VIRTUALLY NO RISK	SLIGHT RISK	MODERATE RISK	STRONG RISK	EXTREME RISK
▓	▓			

Imodium AD is used to treat diarrhea. Studies conducted in rats and rabbits have shown no fetal birth defects after treatment with Imodium AD. One study conducted in humans revealed a small percentage of birth defects in infants exposed to Imodium during the first trimester of pregnancy, including cardiovascular defects. Theses birth defects could have also been caused by other disease states in the mother, or by the use of other drugs. Imodium should be used with some caution during pregnancy.

BREAST-FEEDING: This drug is found in breast milk. The American Academy of Pediatrics considers this drug to be compatible with breast-feeding. As with all drugs, some caution should still be used.

BRAND NAME: **Kaopectate**

GENERIC NAME: **attapulgite**

USES: **To treat diarrhea**

FDA PREGNANCY CATEGORY: **C**

VIRTUALLY NO RISK	SLIGHT RISK	MODERATE RISK	STRONG RISK	EXTREME RISK
▓	▓	▓		

Kaopectate is used to treat diarrhea. According to the manufacturer, there have been no studies conducted to determine its effects on a developing fetus. Kaopectate should be used with caution during pregnancy.

BREAST-FEEDING: This drug is not found in breast milk. Women may breast-feed while taking this drug.

BRAND NAME: **Lotrimin AF**

GENERIC NAME: **clotrimazole**

USES: **To treat ringworm and athlete's foot**

FDA PREGNANCY CATEGORY: **B**

VIRTUALLY NO RISK	SLIGHT RISK	MODERATE RISK	STRONG RISK	EXTREME RISK
▒	▒			

Lotrimin AF is used to treat various topical infections of the skin. It has not been shown to cause birth defects. However, Lotrimin AF should be used with some caution during pregnancy.

BREAST-FEEDING: This drug is not found in breast milk. Women may breast-feed while taking this drug.

BRAND NAME: **Maalox**

GENERIC NAME: **Combination product containing magnesium hydroxide and aluminum hydroxide**

USES: **To treat acid indigestion, heartburn, sour stomach, and upset stomach**

FDA PREGNANCY CATEGORY: **C**

VIRTUALLY NO RISK	SLIGHT RISK	MODERATE RISK	STRONG RISK	EXTREME RISK
▒	▒	▒		

Maalox is used to treat the various symptoms associated with upset stomach and heartburn, both very common problems in pregnancy. Studies conducted in animals have shown no adverse effects with continual use of antacids. However, human studies are limited. All antacids have the potential to interfere with normal iron absorption. Magnesium-containing antacids have the potential to induce diarrhea, and aluminum-containing antacids have the potential to induce constipation. There have been reports of increased muscle tendon problems in the fetuses of mothers who took high doses of antacids for long periods of time during pregnancy. Maalox should be used with caution and only for short periods of time.

BREAST-FEEDING: It is not known whether the drug is found in breast milk. Caution should be used when breast-feeding.

BRAND NAME: **Metamucil**
GENERIC NAME: **psyllium**
Similar to **Citrucel;** see entry for **Citrucel**

BRAND NAME: **Monistat 7**
GENERIC NAME: **miconazole**
USES: **To treat vaginal yeast infections**
FDA PREGNANCY CATEGORY: **C**

VIRTUALLY NO RISK	SLIGHT RISK	MODERATE RISK	STRONG RISK	EXTREME RISK

Monistat 7 is used to treat vaginal fungal infections. A small percentage of infants exposed to Monistat 7 during the first trimester reported major birth defects, including cardiovascular disorders, oral clefts, and defects in the male reproductive organs; however, this limited data does not prove a definite relationship between the use of Monistat 7 and the birth defects. The use of a vaginal applicator may harm the uterus. Monistat 7 should only be used during pregnancy under the close supervision of a physician.

BREAST-FEEDING: It is not known whether the drug is found in breast milk. Some caution should be used when breast-feeding.

BRAND NAME: **Motrin IB**
GENERIC NAME: **ibuprofen**
See entry for **Advil**

BRAND NAME: **Mycelex-7**
GENERIC NAME: **clotrimazole**
See entry for **Gyne-Lotrimin**

BRAND NAME: **Mylanta AR**
GENERIC NAME: **famotidine**
See entry for **Pepcid AC**

BRAND NAME: **Nasalcrom**
GENERIC NAME: **cromolyn sodium**
USES: **For the prevention and relief of nasal allergy symptoms**
FDA PREGNANCY CATEGORY: **B**

VIRTUALLY NO RISK	SLIGHT RISK	MODERATE RISK	STRONG RISK	EXTREME RISK

Nasalcrom is an inhaled drug used for the treatment of nasal allergies and is generally considered safe for use during pregnancy. Although a small percentage of pregnant women treated with Nasalcrom throughout pregnancy have given birth to children with birth defects, no positive association between the drug and birth defects has been established. As with any drug, Nasalcrom should still be used with some caution during pregnancy.

BREAST-FEEDING: It is not known whether the drug is found in breast milk. Caution should be used when breast-feeding.

BRAND NAME: **Neosporin**

GENERIC NAME: **Combination product containing neomycin, bacitracin, and polymyxin B**

USES: **A topical preparation to help prevent infection in minor cuts and scrapes**

FDA PREGNANCY CATEGORY: **C**

VIRTUALLY NO RISK	SLIGHT RISK	MODERATE RISK	STRONG RISK	EXTREME RISK

Neosporin is an antibiotic that is applied topically to the skin and contains three active ingredients—neomycin, bacitracin, and polymyxin B. No reports of birth defects caused by the use of bacitracin in pregnant women are available. In one study, 18 infants were exposed to bacitracin during the first trimester, and no birth defects were reported. Neomycin is an antibiotic that has the potential to cause toxicity to one of the cranial nerves within the fetus. Birth defects caused by the use of polymyxin B have not been reported. In one very small study, seven infants exposed to polymyxin during the first trimester had no birth defects. The product Polysporin is better choice for use during pregnancy because it does not contain neomycin.

BREAST-FEEDING: This drug is not found in breast milk. Women may breast-feed while taking this drug.

BRAND NAME: **Nicoderm CQ**

GENERIC NAME: **nicotine**

USES: **To aid in smoking cessation**

FDA PREGNANCY CATEGORY: **D**

VIRTUALLY NO RISK	SLIGHT RISK	MODERATE RISK	STRONG RISK	EXTREME RISK

The effects of using nicotine skin patches during pregnancy are not entirely known. However, nicotine use in the last trimester of pregnancy has been shown to decrease fetal breathing due to a decrease in blood flow. Miscarriage has also been reported when nicotine is used during pregnancy. The use of nicotine patches should only be considered when the probability of stopping smoking very significantly outweighs the potential harm to the fetus if the mother would continue to smoke. Consultation with a physician is highly recommended.

BREAST-FEEDING: This drug is found in breast milk and may be harmful to a breast-feeding infant. This product should not be used by nursing mothers.

BRAND NAME: **Nicorette Gum**
GENERIC NAME: **nicotine polacrilex**
USES: **To aid in smoking cessation**
FDA PREGNANCY CATEGORY: **D**

VIRTUALLY NO RISK	SLIGHT RISK	MODERATE RISK	STRONG RISK	EXTREME RISK

The effects of using nicotine gum during pregnancy are not entirely known. However, nicotine use in the last trimester of pregnancy has been shown to decrease fetal breathing due to a decrease in blood flow. Miscarriage has also been reported when nicotine is used during pregnancy. The use of nicotine gum should only be considered when the probability of stopping smoking very significantly outweighs the potential harm to the fetus if the mother would continue to smoke. Consultation with a physician is highly recommended.

BREAST-FEEDING: This drug is found in breast milk and may be harmful to a breast-feeding infant. Nursing mothers should not use this product.

BRAND NAME: **Nicotrol NS**

GENERIC NAME: **nicotine**

See entry for **Nicoderm CQ**

BRAND NAME: **Nix**

GENERIC NAME: **permethrin**

USES: **For the treatment of head lice**

FDA PREGNANCY CATEGORY: **B**

VIRTUALLY NO RISK	SLIGHT RISK	MODERATE RISK	STRONG RISK	EXTREME RISK
░░░░░	░░░░░	░░░░░		

Nix is applied topically and used for treatment against various types of lice, ticks, mites, and fleas. No adequate and well-controlled studies have been conducted in pregnant women to determine if Nix has any adverse effects on the fetus. Nix should be used with caution during pregnancy.

BREAST-FEEDING: This drug is found in breast milk. The potential effects of exposure to this drug on a breast-feeding infant are not known. Nursing mothers taking this drug should use extreme caution when breast-feeding.

BRAND NAME: **Nuprin**

GENERIC NAME: **ibuprofen**

See entry for **Advil**

BRAND NAME: **NyQuil**

GENERIC NAME: **Combination product containing pseudoephedrine, doxylamine, acetaminophen, and dextromethorphan**

USES: **To treat cold and flu symptoms**

FDA PREGNANCY CATEGORY: **C**

VIRTUALLY NO RISK	SLIGHT RISK	MODERATE RISK	STRONG RISK	EXTREME RISK

Nyquil is used to help induce sleep and relieve the symptoms associated with colds and flu. It contains four active ingredients—pseudoephedrine, doxylamine, acetaminophen, and dextromethorphan. Pseudoephedrine has been shown to cause birth defects in animals. Exposure to pseudoephedrine during the first trimester has shown a significantly increased risk of fetal malformations. Many physicians suggest avoiding pseudoephedrine during the first trimester of pregnancy and using some caution during the second and third trimesters. The use of doxylamine in combination with other drugs has been associated with birth defects when infants were exposed during the first trimester. Some of these birth defects included abnormalities within the skeleton, limbs, and cardiovascular system. A more significant abnormality—disorders within the valves of the stomach—has also been reported. The use of dextromethorphan in animals has not been studied. However, in one study conducted in humans, an increased risk of congenital birth defects was seen when infants were exposed to dextromethorphan during the first trimester. However, the number of malformations was not great enough to establish a positive relationship between the use of dextromethorphan and the birth defects. Acetaminophen (Tylenol®) is generally considered safe for use during all trimesters of pregnancy for short-term pain relief and fever reduction. Unlike aspirin, acetaminophen does not interfere with platelet function and therefore does not cause a problem with bleeding when given near delivery. The use of NyQuil is not recommended during pregnancy unless its benefits outweigh its potential risks to the fetus.

BRAND NAME: **Nytol**

GENERIC NAME: **diphenhydramine**

See entry for **Benadryl**

BRAND NAME: **Orudis KT**

GENERIC NAME: **ketoprofen**

USES: **To treat mild to moderate pain and inflammation**

FDA PREGNANCY CATEGORY: **B**

VIRTUALLY NO RISK	SLIGHT RISK	MODERATE RISK	STRONG RISK	EXTREME RISK

Orudis is used to treat pain and inflammation. Studies conducted in mice, rats, rabbits, and monkeys have shown no fetal abnormalities. A very small percentage of infants exposed to Orudis during the first trimester had major birth defects, including cardiovascular and limb defects. It should absolutely never be taken during the third trimester because of a possibility of causing high blood pressure in the lungs of the fetus. Inhibition of labor and longer pregnancies have also been associated with the use of Orudis during the third trimester. Women who are trying to become pregnant should avoid Orudis because animal studies indicate the drug may prevent the fertilized egg from implanting in the uterus properly. The use of Orudis during pregnancy should only be considered if its benefits outweigh its potential risks to the fetus.

BREAST-FEEDING: It is not known whether the drug is found in breast milk. Caution should be used when breast-feeding.

BRAND NAME: **Oxy-10**

GENERIC NAME: **benzoyl peroxide 10%**

USES: **To treat acne**

FDA PREGNANCY CATEGORY: **C**

VIRTUALLY NO RISK	SLIGHT RISK	MODERATE RISK	STRONG RISK	EXTREME RISK
▓	▓	▓		

Oxy-10 is a topical product applied to the skin for the treatment of acne. It is not known whether Oxy-10 causes harm to the fetus if used during pregnancy. It should be used with caution during pregnancy.

BREAST-FEEDING: It is not known whether the drug is found in breast milk. Caution should be used when breast-feeding.

BRAND NAME: **Pepcid AC**

GENERIC NAME: **famotidine**

USES: **For prevention and relief of heartburn, acid indigestion, and sour stomach**

FDA PREGNANCY CATEGORY: **B**

VIRTUALLY NO RISK	SLIGHT RISK	MODERATE RISK	STRONG RISK	EXTREME RISK
▓				

Pepcid is used to block the production of excess stomach acid. In rats and rabbits given oral doses greater than 2,000mg, no fetal abnormalities were reported. There are no published reports documenting the use of Pepcid in human pregnancy. However, famotidine is believed to cross the placenta. Pepcid AC should be used with some caution during pregnancy.

BREAST-FEEDING: This drug is found in breast milk. The potential effects of exposure to this drug on a breast-feeding infant are not known. Nursing mothers taking this drug should use caution when breast-feeding.

BRAND NAME: **Pepto-Bismol**

GENERIC NAME: **bismuth subsalicylate**

USES: **To treat diarrhea, stomach cramps, heartburn, and acid indigestion, nausea, and upset stomach**

FDA PREGNANCY CATEGORY: **C**

VIRTUALLY NO RISK	SLIGHT RISK	MODERATE RISK	STRONG RISK	EXTREME RISK

Pepto-Bismol is used to treat diarrhea and stomach upset. Pepto-Bismol is broken down in the gastrointestinal tract into bismuth salts and sodium salicylate. Although only a small percentage of bismuth salts are absorbed, studies in lambs revealed abnormally stunted growth and miscarriage when exposed to this drug over a long period of time. No reports concerning the use of bismuth subsalicylate in pregnancy are available. The salicylate component is very similar to aspirin and is absorbed rapidly. In general, long-term use of salicylates should be avoided at any time during pregnancy. Salicylates can increase the risk of significant bleeding in the fetus anytime during pregnancy. During the last trimester, salicylates may cause heart abnormalities in the fetus. Salicylates absolutely should never be used during the last three months of pregnancy. Pepto-Bismol should be used with extreme caution during the first six months of pregnancy as well.

BREAST-FEEDING: This drug is found in breast milk and may be harmful to a breast-feeding infant. Nursing mothers should not take this drug.

BRAND NAME: **Perdiem**

GENERIC NAME: **psyllium**

Similar to **Citrucel;** see entry for **Citrucel**

BRAND NAME: **Peri-Colace**

GENERIC NAME: **Combination product containing casanthranol and docusate**

See entry for **Doxidan**

BRAND NAME: **Phazyme**

GENERIC NAME: **simethicone**

See entry for **Gas-X**

BRAND NAME: **Phillip's Milk of Magnesia**

GENERIC NAME: **magnesium hydroxide**

USES: **Constipation, acid indigestion, heartburn, and sour stomach**

FDA PREGNANCY CATEGORY: **C**

VIRTUALLY NO RISK	SLIGHT RISK	MODERATE RISK	STRONG RISK	EXTREME RISK

Phillip's Milk of Magnesia is used to treat the various symptoms associated with upset stomach, constipation, and heartburn. Studies conducted in animals have shown no adverse effects when constant administration of antacids occurred. Human studies are limited. All antacids have the potential to interfere with normal iron absorption. Magnesium-containing antacids have the potential to induce diarrhea. There have been reports of imbalances in magnesium and muscle tendon problems in the fetuses of mothers who took high doses of antacids during pregnancy. Phillip's Milk of Magnesia should be used with caution during pregnancy.

BREAST-FEEDING: It is not known whether the drug is found in breast milk. Caution should be used when breast-feeding.

BRAND NAME: **Preparation H Ointment**

GENERIC NAME: **Combination product containing phenylephrine and petrolatum**

USES: **To treat hemorrhoids**

FDA PREGNANCY CATEGORY: **C**

VIRTUALLY NO RISK	SLIGHT RISK	MODERATE RISK	STRONG RISK	EXTREME RISK
▒	▒	▒		

Preparation H is used to treat the pain and inflammation associated with hemorrhoids. It contains two ingredients—phenylephrine and petrolatum. Phenylephrine is used to constrict blood vessels and does have the potential to constrict the blood vessels of the uterus as well. This constriction of blood vessels could decrease oxygen delivery to the fetus. Phenylephrine has been shown to cause birth defects in animals. In humans, several birth defects have been reported after exposure to phenylephrine during the first trimester of pregnancy. Some of these birth defects include eye and ear defects, clubfoot, and fusion of the fingers and toes. Petrolatum is a base in which the phenylephrine is dissolved to make an ointment. The use of Preparation H is not recommended during pregnancy unless its benefits outweigh its potential risks to the fetus.

BREAST-FEEDING: It is not known whether the drug is found in breast milk. Caution should be used when breast-feeding.

BRAND NAME: **Primatene Mist Inhaler**

GENERIC NAME: **epinephrine**

USES: **To treat shortness of breath, tightness of the chest, and wheezing due to asthma**

FDA PREGNANCY CATEGORY: **C**

VIRTUALLY NO RISK	SLIGHT RISK	MODERATE RISK	STRONG RISK	EXTREME RISK
▒	▒	▒		

Primatene is an inhaled drug used to alleviate the symptoms associated with asthma. Epinephrine, the active component of Primatene, is a naturally occurring chemical in the human body. Studies have shown that epinephrine causes birth defects in animals. In one human study, a significant association was found between exposure to epinephrine during the first trimester and fetal malformations, including hernias. Epinephrine has the potential to decrease blood flow to the uterus by constricting blood vessels. This constriction could decrease oxygen delivery to the fetus. Primatene is not recommended for use during pregnancy unless its benefits outweigh its potential risks to the fetus.

BREAST-FEEDING: It is not known whether the drug is found in breast milk. Caution should be used when breast-feeding.

BRAND NAME: **Robitussin DM**
GENERIC NAME: **Combination product containing dextromethorphan and guaifenesin**
USES: **To treat cough**
FDA PREGNANCY CATEGORY: **C**

VIRTUALLY NO RISK	SLIGHT RISK	MODERATE RISK	STRONG RISK	EXTREME RISK

Robitussin DM is used to alleviate coughing and break up mucous. The two active ingredients are dextromethorphan and guaifenesin. The use of dextromethorphan in animals has not been studied. However, in one study conducted in humans, an increased risk of congenital malformations was seen when infants were exposed to dextromethorphan during the first trimester. The number of malformations was not great enough to establish a positive relationship between the use of dextromethorphan and the birth defects. Several studies conducted concerning the use of guaifenesin during the first trimester of pregnancy have shown an increased number of fetal hernias, cardiovascular defects, and abnormal limb formation, but the data do not prove that guaifenesin caused the birth defects. However, caution should still be exercised when considering this drug during pregnancy. Robitussin DM is not recommended for use during pregnancy unless its benefits outweigh its potential risks to the fetus.

BREAST-FEEDING: It is not known whether the drug is found in breast milk. Caution should be used when breast-feeding.

BRAND NAME: **Senokot**
GENERIC NAME: **senna**
See entry for **Ex-Lax**

BRAND NAME: **Sine-Aid**
GENERIC NAME: **Combination product containing acetaminophen and pseudoephedrine**
See entry for **Tylenol® Sinus**

BRAND NAME: **Sinutab**
GENERIC NAME: **Combination product containing acetaminophen, chlorpheniramine, and pseudoephedrine**
See entry for **Theraflu**

BRAND NAME: **Solarcaine**
GENERIC NAME: **benzocaine**
USES: **To treat sunburn and provide topical pain relief**
FDA PREGNANCY CATEGORY: **C**

VIRTUALLY NO RISK	SLIGHT RISK	MODERATE RISK	STRONG RISK	EXTREME RISK

Solarcaine is applied to the skin to relieve the pain and burning associated with sunburn. Safety for use during pregnancy has not been established. Most times sunburn should be left untreated. The use of Solarcaine is not recommended during pregnancy unless its benefits outweigh its potential risks to the fetus.

BREAST-FEEDING: It is not known whether the drug is found in breast milk. Caution should be used when breast-feeding.

BRAND NAME: **Sominex**
GENERIC NAME: **diphenhydramine**
See entry for **Benadryl**

BRAND NAME: **Sudafed**
GENERIC NAME: **pseudoephedrine**
USES: **To treat nasal congestion due to cold or allergy**
FDA PREGNANCY CATEGORY: **C**

VIRTUALLY NO RISK	SLIGHT RISK	MODERATE RISK	STRONG RISK	EXTREME RISK

Sudafed is used to relieve congestion associated with allergies and colds. Pseudoephedrine has been shown to cause birth defects in animals. Exposure to pseudoephedrine during the first trimester has shown a significantly increased risk of fetal malformations in humans. Many physicians suggest avoiding pseudoephedrine during the first trimester of pregnancy and using some caution during the second and third trimesters.

BREAST-FEEDING: This drug is found in breast milk. The American Academy of Pediatrics considers this drug to be compatible with breast-feeding. As with all drugs, some caution should still be taken.

BRAND NAME: **Surfak**

GENERIC NAME: **docusate calcium**

See entry for **Colace**

BRAND NAME: **Tagamet HB**

GENERIC NAME: **cimetidine**

USES: **For the prevention and relief of heartburn, acid indigestion, and sour stomach**

FDA PREGNANCY CATEGORY: **B**

VIRTUALLY NO RISK	SLIGHT RISK	MODERATE RISK	STRONG RISK	EXTREME RISK

Tagamet is used to block the effects of excess stomach acid. It has been shown to cross the placenta. In studies conducted on animals, no evidence of birth defects has been observed in most animals. However, Tagamet has been shown to cause specific adverse effects in male animal offspring. These abnormalities include decreased weight of the testes, prostate gland, and seminal vesicles. All of these organs are necessary for proper reproduction in males. Male animals exposed to Tagamet have also shown decreased levels of the male hormone, testosterone, decreased sexual motivation, and decreased sexual performance. The use of Tagamet in humans has not been proven to cause birth defects; however, isolated cases of heart disease, mental retardation, and clubfoot have occurred. Tagamet is not recommended for use during pregnancy unless its benefits significantly outweigh its potential risks to the fetus.

BREAST-FEEDING: This drug is found in breast milk. The American Academy of Pediatrics considers this drug to be compatible with breast-feeding. As with all drugs, some caution should still be taken.

BRAND NAME: **Tavist-D**

GENERIC NAME: **Combination product containing clemastine and pseudoephedrine**

USES: **To treat nasal congestion due to cold or allergy**

FDA PREGNANCY CATEGORY: **C**

VIRTUALLY NO RISK	SLIGHT RISK	MODERATE RISK	STRONG RISK	EXTREME RISK

Tavist-D is used to relieve symptoms caused by allergies and the common cold. Tavist-D has two active ingredients—clemastine and pseudoephedrine. Pseudoephedrine is used to relieve congestion associated with allergies and colds. It has been shown to cause birth defects in some animals. Exposure to pseudoephedrine during the first trimester has shown a significantly increased risk of fetal malformations. Many physicians suggest avoiding pseudoephedrine during the first trimester of pregnancy and to use some caution during the second and third trimesters. The use of clemastine has been studied in rats and rabbits with no reports of birth defects being documented. In one human study, 4.4 percent of infants exposed to clemastine during the first trimester had some kind of birth defect. These included cardiovascular disorders, spina bifida, defects in the male reproductive organs, and decreased number of limbs. The use of antihistamines during the last two weeks of pregnancy has been associated with retrolental fibroplasia, a fibrous tissue deposit behind the lens of the eye, causing blindness in some prematurely born infants. Clemastine should never be taken during the last two weeks of pregnancy. Tavist-D is not recommended for use during pregnancy unless its benefits outweigh its potential risks to the fetus.

BREAST-FEEDING: This drug is found in breast milk and may be harmful to a breast-feeding infant. This drug should not be taken by nursing mothers.

BRAND NAME: **Theraflu**

GENERIC NAME: **Combination product containing acetaminophen, pseudoephedrine, and chlorpheniramine**

USES: **Relief of cold and flu symptoms**

FDA PREGNANCY CATEGORY: **C**

VIRTUALLY NO RISK	SLIGHT RISK	MODERATE RISK	STRONG RISK	EXTREME RISK

Theraflu is used to relieve the various symptoms associated with the common cold or the flu. Theraflu contains three active ingredients—pseudoephedrine, acetaminophen, and chlorpheniramine. Pseudoephedrine has been shown to cause birth defects in animals. Exposure to pseudoephedrine during the first trimester has shown a significantly increased risk of fetal malformations. Many physicians suggest avoiding pseudoephedrine during the first trimester of pregnancy and using some caution during the second and third trimesters. Acetaminophen (Tylenol®) is generally considered safe for use during all trimesters of pregnancy for short-term pain relief and fever reduction. Unlike aspirin, acetaminophen does not interfere with platelet function and therefore does not cause a problem with bleeding when given near delivery. Birth defects caused by the use of chlorpheniramine during pregnancy have not been proven; however, some malformations have been reported following exposure during pregnancy, including gastrointestinal disorders, hernias, hip dislocations, and eye and ear defects. The use of antihistamines during the last two weeks of pregnancy has been associated with retrolental fibroplasia, a fibrous tissue deposit behind the lens of the eye, causing blindness in some prematurely born infants. Chlorpheniramine should never be used during the last two weeks of pregnancy. Theraflu is not recommended for use during pregnancy unless its benefits outweigh its potential risks to the fetus.

BREAST-FEEDING: It is not known whether the drug is found in breast milk. Caution should be used when breast-feeding.

BRAND NAME: **Tinactin**

GENERIC NAME: **tolnaftate**

USES: **To treat athlete's foot and ringworm**

FDA PREGNANCY CATEGORY: **C**

VIRTUALLY NO RISK	SLIGHT RISK	MODERATE RISK	STRONG RISK	EXTREME RISK
▓▓▓▓	▓▓▓▓	▓▓▓▓		

Tinactin is applied topically in the treatment of athlete's foot or ringworm. According to the manufacturer, no clinical studies have been conducted to determine its effects on a fetus during pregnancy. A small amount may be absorbed into the bloodstream, but is most likely not enough to cause harm to the fetus. However, due to the lack of clinical data, tolnaftate should be used with some caution during pregnancy.

BREAST-FEEDING: This drug is not found in breast milk. Women may breast-feed while taking this drug.

BRAND NAME: **Tums**

GENERIC NAME: **calcium carbonate**

USES: **Heartburn, acid indigestion, and sour stomach**

FDA PREGNANCY CATEGORY: **B**

VIRTUALLY NO RISK	SLIGHT RISK	MODERATE RISK	STRONG RISK	EXTREME RISK
▓▓▓▓	▓▓▓▓			

Tums is used to relieve the symptoms associated with upset stomach and heartburn. The active ingredient, calcium carbonate, is generally safe if given late in the third trimester. No adequate studies in humans are available to determine if Tums has an adverse effect on the developing fetus at other times during pregnancy. Tums should be used with some caution during pregnancy.

BREAST-FEEDING: This drug is not found in breast milk. Women may breast-feed while taking this drug.

BRAND NAME: **Tylenol®**

GENERIC NAME: **acetaminophen**

USES: **To treat mild to moderate pain**

FDA PREGNANCY CATEGORY: **C**

VIRTUALLY NO RISK	SLIGHT RISK	MODERATE RISK	STRONG RISK	EXTREME RISK
░░░░░░░░	░░░░░░░░			

Acetaminophen (Tylenol®) is generally considered safe for use during all trimesters of pregnancy for short-term pain relief and fever reduction. Unlike aspirin, acetaminophen does not interfere with platelet function and therefore does not cause a problem with bleeding when given near to the time of delivery. As with any drug taken during pregnancy, some caution should still be used.

BREAST-FEEDING: This drug is found in breast milk. The American Academy of Pediatrics considers this drug to be compatible with breast-feeding. As with all drugs, some caution should still be used.

BRAND NAME: **Tylenol® Cold and Flu**

GENERIC NAME: **Combination product containing acetaminophen, pseudoephedrine, and dextromethorphan**

USES: **To treat nasal congestion, sore throat, cough, and pain related to the common cold**

FDA PREGNANCY CATEGORY: **C**

VIRTUALLY NO RISK	SLIGHT RISK	MODERATE RISK	STRONG RISK	EXTREME RISK
░░░░░░░░	░░░░░░░░	░░░░░░░░		

Tylenol® Cold and Flu is a combination drug used to treat the various symptoms of the common cold and flu. There are three major ingredients in this product—acetaminophen, pseudoephedrine, and dextromethorphan. Acetaminophen (Tylenol®) is generally considered safe for use during all trimesters of pregnancy for short-term pain relief and fever reduction. Unlike aspirin, acetaminophen does not interfere with platelet function and therefore does not cause a problem with bleeding when given near to the time of delivery. The use of dextromethorphan in animals has not been studied. However, in one study conducted in humans, an increased risk of congenital malformations was seen when infants were exposed to dextromethorphan during the first trimester. The number of malformations was not great enough to establish a positive relationship between the use of dextromethorphan and the birth defects. Pseudoephedrine has been shown to cause birth defects in animals. Exposure to pseudoephedrine during the first trimester has shown a significantly increased risk of fetal malformations. Many physicians suggest avoiding pseudoephedrine during the first trimester of pregnancy and using some caution during the second and third trimesters. Tylenol® Cold and Flu should be used with caution during pregnancy.

BREAST-FEEDING: It is not known whether the drug is found in breast milk. Caution should be used when breast-feeding.

BRAND NAME: **Tylenol® PM**
GENERIC NAME: **Combination product containing acetaminophen and diphenhydramine**
USES: **To treat mild to moderate pain accompanied by insomnia**
FDA PREGNANCY CATEGORY: **C**

VIRTUALLY NO RISK	SLIGHT RISK	MODERATE RISK	STRONG RISK	EXTREME RISK

Tylenol® PM is used to relieve pain and induce sleep. The two active ingredients are acetaminophen and diphenhydramine. Acetaminophen (Tylenol®) is generally considered safe for use during all trimesters of pregnancy for short-term pain relief and fever reduction. Unlike aspirin, acetaminophen does not interfere with platelet function and therefore does not cause a problem with bleeding when given near to the time of delivery. Rats and rabbits who received doses of diphenhydramine of up to 5 times the normal human dose showed no fetal harm. However, some studies have reported birth defects, including hernias, cardiovascular disorders, urinary abnormalities, and eye and ear defects. It has also been shown to cause some uterine contractions. No direct relationship between the use of diphenhydramine and these birth defects has been proven. Abnormalities could have been a result of the mother's disease and the use of other drugs. The use of antihistamines during the last two weeks of pregnancy has been associated with retrolental fibroplasia, a fibrous tissue deposit behind the lens of the eye, causing blindness in some prematurely born infants. Diphenhydramine should never be used during the last two weeks of pregnancy. Tylenol® PM is not recommended for use during pregnancy unless its benefits outweigh its potential risks to the fetus.

BREAST-FEEDING: This drug is found in breast milk and may be harmful to a breast-feeding infant. This drug should not be taken by nursing mothers.

BRAND NAME: **Tylenol® Sinus**
GENERIC NAME: **Combination product containing acetaminophen and pseudoephedrine**
USES: **To treat nasal congestion**
FDA PREGNANCY CATEGORY: **C**

VIRTUALLY NO RISK	SLIGHT RISK	MODERATE RISK	STRONG RISK	EXTREME RISK

Tylenol® Sinus is used to relieve pain associated with cold and allergic disorders. It contains two active ingredients—pseudoephedrine and acetaminophen. Pseudoephedrine has been shown to cause birth defects in animals. Exposure to pseudoephedrine during the first trimester has shown a significantly increased risk of fetal malformations. Many physicians suggest avoiding pseudoephedrine during the first trimester of pregnancy and using some caution during the second and third trimesters. Acetaminophen (Tylenol®) is generally considered safe for use during all trimesters of pregnancy for short-term pain relief and fever reduction. Unlike aspirin, acetaminophen does not interfere with platelet function and therefore does not cause a problem with bleeding when given near to the time of delivery. Tylenol® Sinus should be used with some caution during pregnancy.

BREAST-FEEDING: This drug is found in breast milk. The American Academy of Pediatrics considers this drug to be compatible with breast-feeding. As with all drugs, some caution should still be used.

BRAND NAME: **Unisom**
GENERIC NAME: **doxylamine**
USES: **As a sleep aid**
FDA PREGNANCY CATEGORY: **C**

VIRTUALLY NO RISK	SLIGHT RISK	MODERATE RISK	STRONG RISK	EXTREME RISK

Unisom is used to induce sleep. The use of Unisom in combination with other drugs has been associated with birth defects when infants were exposed during the first trimester. Some of the observed birth defects included abnormalities within the skeleton, limbs, and cardiovascular system. A more significant abnormality was the report of disorders within the valves of the stomach. Unisom is not recommended for use during pregnancy unless its benefits outweigh its potential risks to the fetus.

BREAST-FEEDING: It is not known whether the drug is found in breast milk. Caution should be used when breast-feeding.

BRAND NAME: **Vagistat-1**

GENERIC NAME: **tioconazole**

USES: **To treat yeast infection**

FDA PREGNANCY CATEGORY: **C**

VIRTUALLY NO RISK	SLIGHT RISK	MODERATE RISK	STRONG RISK	EXTREME RISK
░░░░░				

Vagistat-1 is used to treat vaginal fungal infections. No reported birth defects have been associated with its use during pregnancy. Although this drug is applied in the vagina, some of the drug is absorbed into the bloodstream. The use of a vaginal applicator may cause harm to the uterus. Vagistat-1 should only be used during pregnancy under the direct supervision of a physician.

BREAST-FEEDING: It is not known whether the drug is found in breast milk. Some caution should be used when breast-feeding.

BRAND NAME: **Vicks 44D**

GENERIC NAME: **Combination product containing dextromethorphan and pseudoephedrine**

USES: **To treat cough and nasal congestion due to cold**

FDA PREGNANCY CATEGORY: **C**

VIRTUALLY NO RISK	SLIGHT RISK	MODERATE RISK	STRONG RISK	EXTREME RISK
░░░░░	░░░░░	░░░░░		

Vicks 44D is used to relieve symptoms associated with the common cold and to suppress cough. Vicks 44D has two active ingredients—pseudoephedrine and dextromethorphan. Pseudoephedrine has been shown to cause birth defects in animals. Exposure to pseudoephedrine during the first trimester has shown a significantly increased risk of fetal malformations. Many physicians suggest avoiding pseudoephedrine during the first trimester of pregnancy and using some caution during the second and third trimesters. The use of dextromethorphan in animals has not been studied. However, in one study conducted in humans, an increased risk of congenital malformations was seen when infants were exposed to dextromethorphan during the first trimester. The number of malformations was not great enough to establish a positive relationship between the use of dextromethorphan and the birth defects. These reports do not confirm a definite relationship between the use of pseudoephedrine and birth defects. Vicks 44D is not recommended during pregnancy unless its benefits outweigh its potential risks to the fetus.

BREAST-FEEDING: It is not known whether the drug is found in breast milk. Caution should be used when breast-feeding.

BRAND NAME: **Zantac 75**
GENERIC NAME: **ranitidine**
USES: **To treat gastric ulcer, gastroesophageal reflux disease (GERD), and heartburn**
FDA PREGNANCY CATEGORY: **B**

VIRTUALLY NO RISK	SLIGHT RISK	MODERATE RISK	STRONG RISK	EXTREME RISK

Zantac is used to block the effects of excess stomach acid. It has been shown to cross the placenta. In studies conducted in rats and rabbits, no birth defects have been reported. An observational study looking at the effects of first-trimester exposure to Zantac showed only a small percentage of birth defects, including cardiovascular defects, spina bifida, and hypospadias, a defect in the penis of male offspring. This small percentage of birth defects does not prove a direct relationship between the use of Zantac and these birth defects. Zantac should be used with some caution during pregnancy.

BREAST-FEEDING: This drug is found in breast milk. The potential effects of exposure to this drug on a breast-feeding infant are not known. Nursing mothers taking this drug should use caution when breast-feeding.

CHAPTER 4

Herbal and Homeopathic Products

Herbal products, homeopathic products, and dietary supplements are currently the fastest growing category of products in drugstores. There are over 500 herbal and homeopathic products currently on the market. In 1999, over $3.5 billion was spent on herbal products and dietary supplements in pharmacies, a 60 percent increase in five years. Consumers also spent several billion more in health food stores. This exponential growth in the use of herbal and homeopathic products is expected to continue well into the next century as consumers seek alternative treatments to traditional drug therapy. Consumers tend to view these products as extremely safe because they come from natural or organic sources, such as plants, roots, leaves, and flowers. Prescription drugs like Lanoxin for heart arrhythmias and Taxol for cancer also come from natural sources as well. But these drugs are extremely dangerous and can be very toxic unless prescribed and administered by competent health care practitioners. Therefore, consumers must realize that any foreign product, substance, or chemical placed into the body does have the potential to cause serious harm. Herbal and homeopathic products and dietary supplements are no exception.

Many consumers do not realize that herbal and homeopathic products are virtually unregulated by the Food and Drug Administration (FDA), the federal agency that regulates prescription and over-the-counter drugs. These products are classified by the FDA as foods or dietary supplements. This means that herbal products do not have to go through the rigorous testing that prescription and even over-the-counter medications do. Herbal products do not have to prove that they are either safe or effective in the diseases and conditions they claim to treat. As a trade-off to being classified as a food or dietary supplement, these products cannot make any therapeutic claims or claim to specifically treat certain medical conditions. To get around this legal requirement, many products use very broad or generic therapeutic claims such as "supports healthy living," "promotes cardiovascular health," and "aids in the maintenance of a healthy immune system." These are called structural function claims. Another potential problem with herbal and homeopathic products is their purity. These products do not have to meet any sort of minimum purity standards. Therefore, the actual concentration in any given product may vary by as much as 50 to 500 percent. The loose regulation of these products, the lack of controlled studies regarding their safety and effectiveness, and the relatively short amount of time many of these products have been used causes many doctors and pharmacists to question their safety and effectiveness.

In early 2000, the FDA fought to keep broad therapeutic claims regarding pregnancy off the labels of these products. This battle is still being fought. The FDA, however, has adopted a specific position. They believe that, with the exception of vitamins and minerals that are used to prevent deficiency states, dietary supplements and herbal products should not be used during pregnancy due to the lack of safety information about their use during pregnancy. Furthermore, the FDA believes that all herbal and homeopathic products and dietary supplements should bear the following warning: "Women of childbearing age should consult with a physician before taking this product because dietary supplements are exempt from many aspects of FDA oversight." The FDA does realize, however, that there are certain classes of products that may be beneficial. These products are mostly vitamin and mineral formulations.

The information provided below represents what is currently known about the most popular herbal and homeopathic products and their use in pregnant women. The FDA has not given any of these products a pregnancy category classification because they are not considered drug products. Therefore, no such classification or categorization is provided for each drug. However, based on the current medical literature, risk ratings were assigned.

Finally, the information for each product may seemed somewhat limited and general in nature. Very little is known about the effects and safety of these products in women who are pregnant. Because so little is known, expectant mothers should always use extreme caution before using any of these products. Always consult your doctor and/or pharmacist before taking any herbal remedy, dietary supplement, or homeopathic product.

COMMON NAME: **Aloe**
PROPER NAME: **Aloe barbadensis**
OTHER NAMES: **Lily of the desert, elephant's gall, burn plant**
USES: **As a laxative, to treat seizures, asthma, ulcers, and bleeding, and for many other purposes**
FDA PREGNANCY CATEGORY: **None assigned**

VIRTUALLY NO RISK	SLIGHT RISK	MODERATE RISK	STRONG RISK	EXTREME RISK

This product is most often used as a stimulant laxative when taken internally. It has been shown to be effective for this purpose. However, aloe can potentially cause miscarriage and stimulate contractions in the uterus. Pregnant women should not take this product.

BREAST-FEEDING: This drug is found in breast milk and may be harmful to a breast-feeding infant. This drug should not be taken by nursing mothers.

COMMON NAME: **Bayberry**

PROPER NAME: **Myrica cerifera**

OTHER NAMES: **Candleberry, waxberry, wax myrtle**

USES: **To treat head colds, colitis, diarrhea, and as a circulatory stimulant**

FDA PREGNANCY CATEGORY: **None assigned**

VIRTUALLY NO RISK	SLIGHT RISK	MODERATE RISK	STRONG RISK	EXTREME RISK

The effectiveness of this product has not been demonstrated. The product contains high amounts of tannins, which may be harmful to the fetus. Due to a lack of clinical experience regarding the use of this product during pregnancy, it should be avoided.

BREAST-FEEDING: It is not known whether the product is found in breast milk. Caution should be used when breast-feeding.

COMMON NAME: **Bee Pollen**

PROPER NAME: **None**

OTHER NAMES: **Buckwheat pollen, maize pollen, pine pollen**

USES: **For nutrition, as an appetite stimulant, for improved stamina, for prevention of hay fever or allergic rhinitis**

FDA PREGNANCY CATEGORY: **None assigned**

VIRTUALLY NO RISK	SLIGHT RISK	MODERATE RISK	STRONG RISK	EXTREME RISK

This product is most often used to increase energy or prevent allergies when taken internally. Some studies have shown it to be effective for this purpose. However, bee pollen can potentially stimulate the uterus, which may cause miscarriage and contractions. Pregnant women should not take this product.

BREAST-FEEDING: It is not known whether the product is found in breast milk. Caution should be used when breast-feeding.

COMMON NAME: **Bilberry**
PROPER NAME: **Vaccinium myrtillus**
OTHER NAMES: **Huckleberry, blueberry, wineberry, trackleberry**
USES: **To treat diabetes, arthritis, gout, hemorrhoids, and intestinal diseases**
FDA PREGNANCY CATEGORY: **None assigned**

VIRTUALLY NO RISK	SLIGHT RISK	MODERATE RISK	STRONG RISK	EXTREME RISK

Bilberry has been used to treat several different diseases and health problems. The herb has not been proven effective for any of these uses and is potentially toxic to the fetus. Pregnant women should not take this product.

BREAST-FEEDING: It is not known whether the product is found in breast milk. Caution should be used when breast-feeding.

COMMON NAME: **Black Horehound and Ballota**
PROPER NAME: **Ballota nigra**
OTHER NAMES: **Stinking horehound**
USES: **To treat nausea, vomiting, and for sedation in cases of hysteria and hypochondria**
FDA PREGNANCY CATEGORY: **None assigned**

VIRTUALLY NO RISK	SLIGHT RISK	MODERATE RISK	STRONG RISK	EXTREME RISK

Black horehound has been used to treat nausea and vomiting in pregnant women with morning sickness. Its effectiveness for this use has not been proven. This herb is known to affect the menstrual cycle and may have adverse effects on the uterus during pregnancy. Pregnant women should use extreme caution when taking this product.

BREAST-FEEDING: It is not known whether the product is found in breast milk. Caution should be used when breast-feeding.

COMMON NAME: **Cabbage**
PROPER NAME: **Brassica oleracea**
OTHER NAMES: **Colewort**
USES: **To treat gastritis, gastric or duodenal ulcers, other intestinal disorders, and for breast-feeding problems**
FDA PREGNANCY CATEGORY: **None assigned**

VIRTUALLY NO RISK	SLIGHT RISK	MODERATE RISK	STRONG RISK	EXTREME RISK
▒	▒			

Cabbage has not been proven to be effective in treating any gastro-intestinal-related disorders, nor in assisting in breast-feeding problems, such as increasing milk production. This product is very safe when eaten in normal quantities as part of a well-balanced diet. Cabbage should, however, be avoided in excessive and extremely concentrated amounts because its effects on the fetus are not known.

BREAST-FEEDING: It is not known how much of the product is found in breast milk. Some caution should be used when breast-feeding if excessive or highly concentrated amounts of cabbage extract are used.

COMMON NAME: **Cascara Sagrada**
PROPER NAME: **Rhamnus purshiana**
OTHER NAMES: **Bitter bark, dogwood bark, California buckhorn, yellow bark, and sagrada bark**
USES: **As a laxative, to treat gallstones and liver ailments, and as a bitter tonic**
FDA PREGNANCY CATEGORY: **C**

VIRTUALLY NO RISK	SLIGHT RISK	MODERATE RISK	STRONG RISK	EXTREME RISK
▒	▒	▒		

Cascara is approved by the FDA for short-term use as a laxative. The product should never be used longer than seven days without a physician's approval. The product has been used during pregnancy during the first trimester in a small number of patients. No adverse effects or malformations were found. A larger study found that some fetuses developed benign tumors when the mother used cascara. It was not known whether the drug or something else caused this problem. Pregnant women should use caution when taking this product.

BREAST-FEEDING: This drug is found in breast milk and may cause diarrhea in a breast-feeding infant. This drug should not be taken by nursing mothers.

COMMON NAME: **Chamomile**
PROPER NAME: **Chamaemelum nobile**
OTHER NAMES: **English chamomile, ground apple, Roman chamomile**
USES: **To treat nausea, vomiting, and morning sickness**
FDA PREGNANCY CATEGORY: **None assigned**

VIRTUALLY NO RISK	SLIGHT RISK	MODERATE RISK	STRONG RISK	EXTREME RISK

This product has not been proven effective in treating nausea, vomiting, or morning sickness. Chamomile has also been shown to have some adverse effects on the uterus when using during pregnancy. In extreme cases, the product has the potential to cause miscarriage. Chamomile should be avoiding during pregnancy.

BREAST-FEEDING: It is not known whether the product is found in breast milk. Caution should be used when breast-feeding.

COMMON NAME: **Chickweed**

PROPER NAME: **Stellaria media**

OTHER NAMES: **Star chickweed, starweed**

USES: **To treat constipation, asthma, stomach and bowel problems, obesity, and scurvy**

FDA PREGNANCY CATEGORY: **None assigned**

VIRTUALLY NO RISK	SLIGHT RISK	MODERATE RISK	STRONG RISK	EXTREME RISK

Chickweed is believed to be ineffective for all of the disease states and health problems it claims to treat, and its potential effects on the fetus are unknown; therefore, it should not be used during pregnancy.

BREAST-FEEDING: It is not known whether the product is found in breast milk. Caution should be used when breast-feeding.

COMMON NAME: **Chondroitin**

PROPER NAME: **Chondroitin 4-sulfate**

OTHER NAMES: **Chondroitin Sulfate A, CDS, CSA, CSC**

USES: **To treat osteoarthritis**

FDA PREGNANCY CATEGORY: **None assigned**

VIRTUALLY NO RISK	SLIGHT RISK	MODERATE RISK	STRONG RISK	EXTREME RISK

Many studies have found chondroitin to be effective in treating osteoarthritis. Even though not all scientific experts agree, all of the published studies show positive results. Chondroitin has not been studied in pregnant women and the potential adverse effects on the fetus are unknown. Pregnant women should exercise extreme caution when taking this supplement.

BREAST-FEEDING: It is not known whether the product is found in breast milk. Caution should be used when breast-feeding.

COMMON NAME: **Comfrey**

PROPER NAME: **Symphytum officinale**

OTHER NAMES: **Ass ear, black root, healing herb, slippery root**

USES: **To help heal tears around vaginal opening, to treat ulcers, wounds, and fractures**

FDA PREGNANCY CATEGORY: **None assigned**

VIRTUALLY NO RISK	SLIGHT RISK	MODERATE RISK	STRONG RISK	EXTREME RISK

Comfrey is believed to help treat and possibly prevent tearing around the vaginal opening before and after birth. Its effectiveness when applied topically is questionable at best. It is unknown whether it is safe to use on the vaginal opening during pregnancy, and it is known to be toxic to the liver when taken orally. Therefore, it should be used with caution during pregnancy.

BREAST-FEEDING: It is not known whether the product is found in breast milk. Extreme caution should be used when breast-feeding. However, the chances of topically applied comfrey being found in breast milk are most likely rare.

COMMON NAME: **Dandelion**

PROPER NAME: **Taraxacum officinale**

OTHER NAMES: **Common dandelion, lion's tooth, wild endive**

USES: **To treat loss of appetite, upset stomach, gas, and feeling of fullness in the stomach**

FDA PREGNANCY CATEGORY: **None assigned**

VIRTUALLY NO RISK	SLIGHT RISK	MODERATE RISK	STRONG RISK	EXTREME RISK

When dandelion is consumed in foods and salads, the herb is generally considered safe. It should, however, be avoided in excessive and extremely concentrated amounts because its effect on the fetus is not known.

BREAST-FEEDING: It is not known how much of the product is found in breast milk. Caution should be used when breast-feeding if excessive or highly concentrated amounts of dandelion extract are used.

COMMON NAME: **Dong Quai**
PROPER NAME: **Angelica sinesis**
OTHER NAMES: **Chinese angelica, Dang Gui, Tang Kuei, Dong Qua**
USES: **To treat gynecological ailments, including menstrual cramps, irregularity, weakness during menstrual flow, and other discomforts**
FDA PREGNANCY CATEGORY: **None assigned**

VIRTUALLY NO RISK	SLIGHT RISK	MODERATE RISK	STRONG RISK	EXTREME RISK

In large quantities, Dong Quai is believed to cause cancer and its effectiveness in treating menstrual problems is questionable at best. This drug is considered unsafe for use during pregnancy because of its potential to cause birth defects. It should be avoided at all costs during pregnancy.

BREAST-FEEDING: This product is found in breast milk and may be harmful to a breast-feeding infant. This drug should not be taken by nursing mothers.

COMMON NAME: **Echinacea**
PROPER NAME: **Echinacea angustifolia, Echinacea pallida, E. purpurea**
OTHER NAMES: **Black Susan, scurvy root, snakeroot, American cone flower**
USES: **To treat and prevent colds and other upper-respiratory infections**
FDA PREGNANCY CATEGORY: **None assigned**

VIRTUALLY NO RISK	SLIGHT RISK	MODERATE RISK	STRONG RISK	EXTREME RISK

Echinacea is believed to stimulate the immune system and thus shorten the duration of the common cold. There are some studies that support this claim, but there are no studies regarding its use during pregnancy. It should be avoided unless its potential benefits outweigh its potential risks to the fetus.

BREAST-FEEDING: It is not known whether the product is found in breast milk. Caution should be used when breast-feeding.

COMMON NAME: **Evening Primrose**
PROPER NAME: **Oenothera biennis**
OTHER NAMES: **Fever plant, night willow-herb, King's Cureall**
USES: **To treat PMS, prevent preeclampsia, to treat eczema, psoriasis, and other skin disorders**
FDA PREGNANCY CATEGORY: **None assigned**

VIRTUALLY NO RISK	SLIGHT RISK	MODERATE RISK	STRONG RISK	EXTREME RISK

Evening primrose is sometimes taken to prevent preeclampsia and late delivery dates. For these indications, the drug has been found to be ineffective and should not be taken. It has been found to potentially increase the risk of some complications in pregnancy, including rupture of the membranes in the uterus, slowing the descent of the baby into the birth canal, and increasing the need for vacuum extraction. Evening primrose should be avoided during pregnancy.

BREAST-FEEDING: Evening primrose is found in breast milk and may be harmful to a breast-feeding infant. It should not be taken by nursing mothers.

COMMON NAME: **Feverfew**

PROPER NAME: **Tanacetum parthenium**

OTHER NAMES: **Bachelor's button, featherfew, midsummer daisy**

USES: **To treat fever, migraine headache, menstrual irregularities, and stomachache**

FDA PREGNANCY CATEGORY: **None assigned**

VIRTUALLY NO RISK	SLIGHT RISK	MODERATE RISK	STRONG RISK	EXTREME RISK
▓	▓			

There is some evidence that suggests feverfew may be useful in preventing and treating migraine headaches. However, feverfew is believed to stimulate contractions of the uterus and may cause miscarriage. It therefore should be avoided during pregnancy.

BREAST-FEEDING: It is not known whether the product is found in breast milk. Caution should be used when breast-feeding.

COMMON NAME: **Garlic**

PROPER NAME: **Allium sativum**

OTHER NAMES: **Camphor of the poor, clove garlic, stinking rose**

USES: **To reduce high blood pressure, prevent age-related vascular changes, and lower cholesterol**

FDA PREGNANCY CATEGORY: **None assigned**

VIRTUALLY NO RISK	SLIGHT RISK	MODERATE RISK	STRONG RISK	EXTREME RISK
▓	▓			

Garlic has been proven to lower cholesterol and blood pressure when taken in large quantities. It is very safe when eaten in normal quantities as part of a well-balanced diet. It should, however, be avoided in excessive and extremely concentrated amounts. In large amounts or high doses, garlic may stimulate contractions of the uterus.

BREAST-FEEDING: It is not known how much garlic passes into the breast milk. One study has found that garlic intake by the mother may decrease nursing time by the infant. Some caution should be used when breast-feeding if excessive or highly concentrated amounts of garlic are taken by the nursing mother.

COMMON NAME: **Ginger**
PROPER NAME: **Zingiber officinale**
OTHER NAMES: **African ginger, black ginger, Jamaica ginger**
USES: **To treat motion sickness, morning sickness, colic, upset stomach, arthritis**
FDA PREGNANCY CATEGORY: **None assigned**

VIRTUALLY NO RISK	SLIGHT RISK	MODERATE RISK	STRONG RISK	EXTREME RISK

The effectiveness of the product when used to treat nausea and morning sickness is questionable. Ginger is safe when eaten in normal quantities as part of a well-balanced diet. The product should, however, be avoided in excessive and extremely concentrated amounts. One case of spontaneous abortion was reported by a pregnant woman who was taking large amounts of ginger to prevent morning sickness. Furthermore, the effects of large amounts of ginger on the fetus are unknown.

BREAST-FEEDING: It is not known how much of the product is found in breast milk; therefore extreme caution should be used when breast-feeding if excessive or highly concentrated amounts of ginger are taken by the nursing mother.

COMMON NAME: **Ginkgo or Gingko**
PROPER NAME: **Ginkgo biloba**
OTHER NAMES: **Fossil tree, kew tree, maidenhair tree**
USES: **To improve memory; to treat Alzheimer's disease, asthma, bronchitis, poor circulation, arteriosclerosis**
FDA PREGNANCY CATEGORY: **None assigned**

VIRTUALLY NO RISK	SLIGHT RISK	MODERATE RISK	STRONG RISK	EXTREME RISK

Ginkgo is used by thousands of people in an effort to improve memory. The drug has shown some limited benefits in treating Alzheimer's disease, but has not been proven effective in improving memory. Ginkgo is believed to be potentially harmful to the fetus and may cause birth defects. It should only be used when its benefits greatly outweigh its risks.

BREAST-FEEDING: Ginkgo is found in breast milk and may harm the infant. Nursing mothers should avoid this product while breast-feeding.

COMMON NAME: **Ginseng**
PROPER NAME: **Panax quinquefolius**
OTHER NAMES: **American Ginseng, red berry, Ren Shen**
USES: **As a diuretic, to improve energy, as a digestive aid, and to treat diabetes, fever, insomnia, and hangover symptoms**
FDA PREGNANCY CATEGORY: **None assigned**

VIRTUALLY NO RISK	SLIGHT RISK	MODERATE RISK	STRONG RISK	EXTREME RISK

There is some limited evidence that ginseng may increase endurance, improve stamina, and increase mental alertness. These claims have yet to be proven through rigorous clinical studies. When used during pregnancy, the effects of this product on the fetus are not known, so it should only be used when its benefits outweigh its risks.

BREAST-FEEDING: This product is found in breast milk and has been found to be harmful to a breast-feeding infant. It should never be taken by nursing mothers.

COMMON NAME: **Glucosamine**

PROPER NAME: **2-amino-2-deoxyglucose sulfate**

OTHER NAMES: **Glucosamine sulfate**

USES: **To treat joint inflammation and degeneration**

FDA PREGNANCY CATEGORY: **None assigned**

VIRTUALLY NO RISK	SLIGHT RISK	MODERATE RISK	STRONG RISK	EXTREME RISK

There are a few studies that have found glucosamine is effective in treating osteoarthritis when combined with chondroitin. Even though not all scientific experts agree, some of the published studies show positive results. Glucosamine has not been studied in pregnant women and the potential adverse effects on the fetus are unknown. Women who are pregnant should use caution when taking this product.

BREAST-FEEDING: It is not known whether the product is found in breast milk. Caution should be used when breast-feeding.

COMMON NAME: **Goat's Rue**

PROPER NAME: **Galega officinalis**

OTHER NAMES: **French honeysuckle, French lilac**

USES: **To treat diabetes, as a diuretic, and to increase milk flow**

FDA PREGNANCY CATEGORY: **None assigned**

VIRTUALLY NO RISK	SLIGHT RISK	MODERATE RISK	STRONG RISK	EXTREME RISK

The product is believed to increase milk flow and encourages the development of the breasts, which aids in breast-feeding. Goat's rue has not been proven to be effective for this use. It has not been studied in pregnant women and the potential adverse effects on the fetus are unknown. Pregnant women should use caution when taking this product.

BREAST-FEEDING: It is not known whether the product is found in breast milk. Caution should be used when breast-feeding.

COMMON NAME: **Goldenseal**
PROPER NAME: **Hydrastis canadensis**
OTHER NAMES: **Eye balm, eye root, Indian plant, orange root, turmeric root**
USES: **As a diuretic, to treat diarrhea, to mask the appearance of illegal drugs in a urine test**
FDA PREGNANCY CATEGORY: **None assigned**

VIRTUALLY NO RISK	SLIGHT RISK	MODERATE RISK	STRONG RISK	EXTREME RISK

Some limited research suggests that goldenseal may be somewhat effective in treating mild cases of diarrhea caused by *E. coli* bacteria. It has not been proven effective in masking the detection of illegal drugs in the urine. Goldenseal stimulates the uterus and menstrual cycle and may cause premature contractions. This product should not be used unless its benefits greatly outweigh its risks.

BREAST-FEEDING: It is not known whether the product is found in breast milk. Caution should be used when breast-feeding.

COMMON NAME: **Grape Seed**

PROPER NAME: **Vitis vinifera**

OTHER NAMES: **Grape seed extract, muskat**

USES: **To treat circulatory disorders, varicose veins**

FDA PREGNANCY CATEGORY: **None assigned**

VIRTUALLY NO RISK	SLIGHT RISK	MODERATE RISK	STRONG RISK	EXTREME RISK
▓▓▓				

Grape seed extract contains large amounts of tocopherols (vitamin E). Some patients use this product as a natural vitamin E substitute. The product is safe when eaten in normal quantities as part of a well-balanced diet. The product should, however, be avoided in excessive and extremely concentrated amounts. In large doses, the potential effects on the fetus are unknown. This product should be used with caution in excessive amounts during pregnancy.

BREAST-FEEDING: It is not known whether the product is found in breast milk. Caution should be used when breast-feeding.

COMMON NAME: **Juniper**

PROPER NAME: **Juniperus communis**

OTHER NAMES: **juniper berry, Ginepro, Enebro**

USES: **To treat upset stomach, gas, heartburn, loss of appetite, and urinary tract infections**

FDA PREGNANCY CATEGORY: **None assigned**

VIRTUALLY NO RISK	SLIGHT RISK	MODERATE RISK	STRONG RISK	EXTREME RISK
▓▓▓				

Juniper has not been proven effective in treating any of the above-mentioned conditions. In addition, the product is believed to be unsafe if used for periods longer than four weeks. There is some evidence that juniper can interfere with fertility, affect uterine tone, interfere with implantation of a fertilized egg into the uterus, and potentially cause a miscarriage. Juniper should not be used during pregnancy.

BREAST-FEEDING: It is not known whether the product is found in breast milk. Caution should be used when breast-feeding.

COMMON NAME: **Kava**
PROPER NAME: **Piper methysticum**
OTHER NAMES: **Awa, kava kava, kew, tonga**
USES: **To treat anxiety, stress, and restlessness**
FDA PREGNANCY CATEGORY: **None assigned**

VIRTUALLY NO RISK	SLIGHT RISK	MODERATE RISK	STRONG RISK	EXTREME RISK

There is some evidence that kava may be effective in treating anxiety and restlessness if the product contains 70 percent kavapyrones. However, the product should not be used for more than three months and should definitely not be used during pregnancy. Kava can cause a loss of tone (strength) in the uterus, which may cause bleeding and miscarriage.

BREAST-FEEDING: This product is found in breast milk and has been found to be toxic to a breast-feeding infant. It should not be taken by nursing mothers.

COMMON NAME: **Licorice**
PROPER NAME: **Glycyrrhiza glabra**
OTHER NAMES: **Sweet root, gan cao, Russian licorice**
USES: **To treat upper respiratory tract inflammation, ulcers, bronchitis, colic, upset stomach**
FDA PREGNANCY CATEGORY: **None assigned**

VIRTUALLY NO RISK	SLIGHT RISK	MODERATE RISK	STRONG RISK	EXTREME RISK

There is some limited evidence that licorice may be beneficial in reducing the inflammation in the sinus passages and aid in the healing of ulcers. The product is safe when eaten in small quantities as a food or snack. Licorice should, however, be avoided in excessive and extremely concentrated amounts. Large amounts of licorice can stimulate uterine contractions, mimic the effects of steroids, and potentially cause miscarriage. Large amounts of licorice should be avoided during pregnancy.

BREAST-FEEDING: Licorice is found in breast milk when eaten in large quantities and may cause low potassium and high blood pressure in a breast-fed infant. Large amounts of licorice should be avoided while breast-feeding.

COMMON NAME: **Melatonin**
PROPER NAME: **N-acetyl-5-methoxytryptamine**
OTHER NAMES: **MEL**
USES: **To treat insomnia, jet lag, depression**
FDA PREGNANCY CATEGORY: **None assigned**

VIRTUALLY NO RISK	SLIGHT RISK	MODERATE RISK	STRONG RISK	EXTREME RISK

Some studies have shown that melatonin may be effective in treating jet lag, insomnia, and other types of sleep disorders. It has not been studied in pregnant women, and the potential adverse effects on the fetus are unknown. Women who are pregnant should use caution when taking this product.

BREAST-FEEDING: It is not known whether the product is found in breast milk. Caution should be used when breast-feeding.

COMMON NAME: **Milk Thistle**

PROPER NAME: **Silybum marianum**

OTHER NAMES: **Holy thistle, lady's thistle**

USES: **To treat gallbladder and liver disorders**

FDA PREGNANCY CATEGORY: **None assigned**

VIRTUALLY NO RISK	SLIGHT RISK	MODERATE RISK	STRONG RISK	EXTREME RISK

Milk thistle has not been proven effective in treating gallbladder or liver disorders due to the lack of clinical experience and studies. It has not been studied in pregnant women and the potential adverse effects on the fetus are unknown. Women who are pregnant should use caution when taking this product.

BREAST-FEEDING: It is not known whether the product is found in breast milk. Caution should be used when breast-feeding.

COMMON NAME: **Myrrh**

PROPER NAME: **Commiphora molmol**

OTHER NAMES: **African myrrh, bol, bola, gum myrrh**

USES: **To treat inflamed gums, gingivitis, chapped lips, and other disorders of the mouth and gums**

FDA PREGNANCY CATEGORY: **None assigned**

VIRTUALLY NO RISK	SLIGHT RISK	MODERATE RISK	STRONG RISK	EXTREME RISK

Some limited clinical evidence has found that the product may be effective when applied topically to chapped lips and inflamed gums. Myrrh has not been found to be effective when taken orally for these conditions. The oral form of the product should not be used during pregnancy. It may stimulate uterine contractions, increase blood flow to the uterus, and may cause miscarriage. When used topically in the mouth, the potential adverse effects on the fetus are not known and myrrh therefore should be used with some caution.

BREAST-FEEDING: It is not known whether the product is found in breast milk. Caution should be used when breast-feeding.

COMMON NAME: **Passionflower**
PROPER NAME: **Passiflora incarnata**
OTHER NAMES: **Apricot vine, maypop, passion vine, water lemon**
USES: **To treat anxiety, restlessness, insomnia, and nervous stomach**
FDA PREGNANCY CATEGORY: **None assigned**

VIRTUALLY NO RISK	SLIGHT RISK	MODERATE RISK	STRONG RISK	EXTREME RISK

There is some limited evidence that the product may be effective in treating anxiety and mild insomnia. However, passionflower has been shown to cause uterine contractions and stimulation. It should be avoided during pregnancy.

BREAST-FEEDING: It is not known whether the product is found in breast milk. Caution should be used when breast-feeding.

COMMON NAME: **St. John's-wort**
PROPER NAME: **Hypericum perforatum**
OTHER NAMES: **Johns wort, goatweed, rosin rose, tipton weed**
USES: **To treat depression and anxiety**
FDA PREGNANCY CATEGORY: **None assigned**

VIRTUALLY NO RISK	SLIGHT RISK	MODERATE RISK	STRONG RISK	EXTREME RISK

St. John's-wort has been proven effective in treating depression. In fact, it is the number one prescribed drug for depression in Germany. St.

John's-wort has also been used to speed healing in the perineum after birth but has not been proven effective for this use. St. John's-wort can affect the muscle tone of the uterus. This drug should not be used during pregnancy.

BREAST-FEEDING: It is not known whether the product is found in breast milk. Caution should be used when breast-feeding.

COMMON NAME: **Sassafras**
PROPER NAME: **Sassafras albidum**
OTHER NAMES: **Cinnamon wood, sassafrax, saxifrax**
USES: **To treat urinary problems and to reduce inflammation in mucous membranes**
FDA PREGNANCY CATEGORY: **None assigned**

VIRTUALLY NO RISK	SLIGHT RISK	MODERATE RISK	STRONG RISK	EXTREME RISK

This product has not been proven effective in treating urinary problems or inflammation due to the lack of clinical experience and studies. Sassafras oil should not be used at all during pregnancy owing to its potential to cause miscarriage and uterine bleeding. Pregnant women should avoid drinking sassafras tea as well, even though the chance of the same adverse effects occurring is smaller.

BREAST-FEEDING: It is not known whether the product is found in breast milk. Caution should be used when breast-feeding.

COMMON NAME: **Scullcap**

PROPER NAME: **Scutellaria lateriflora**

OTHER NAMES: **Hoodwort, mad-dog herb, Quaker bonnet, and skullcap**

USES: **To treat insomnia, anxiety, and paralysis caused by a stroke**

FDA PREGNANCY CATEGORY: **None assigned**

VIRTUALLY NO RISK	SLIGHT RISK	MODERATE RISK	STRONG RISK	EXTREME RISK
▒	▒	▒		

There is some limited evidence that the product may be effective in treating paralysis caused by a stroke when given intravenously. However, scullcap has not been proven effective in treating insomnia or anxiety. It has not been studied in pregnant women, and the potential adverse effects on the fetus are unknown. Women who are pregnant should use caution when taking this product.

BREAST-FEEDING: It is not known whether the product is found in breast milk. Caution should be used when breast-feeding.

COMMON NAME: **Tryptophan**

PROPER NAME: **L-Tryptophan**

OTHER NAMES: **L-Tryptophan and L-trypt**

USES: **To treat insomnia and depression**

FDA PREGNANCY CATEGORY: **None assigned**

VIRTUALLY NO RISK	SLIGHT RISK	MODERATE RISK	STRONG RISK	EXTREME RISK
▒	▒	▒	▒	

There is limited evidence that the product may be effective in treating mild insomnia. However, tryptophan has been shown to cause respiratory depression and breathing difficulties in the fetus. It should be avoided during pregnancy.

BREAST-FEEDING: This product is found in breast milk and may be harmful to a breast-feeding infant. It should not be taken by nursing mothers.

COMMON NAME: **Uva Ursi**

PROPER NAME: **Arctostaphylos uva-ursi**

OTHER NAMES: **Bearberry, bearsgrape, hogberry, rockberry, and sandberry**

USES: **To treat urinary problems**

FDA PREGNANCY CATEGORY: **None assigned**

VIRTUALLY NO RISK	SLIGHT RISK	MODERATE RISK	STRONG RISK	EXTREME RISK

There is limited evidence that the product may be effective in treating inflammatory problems in the urinary tract. However, uva ursi should only be used for very short periods of time. It may be unsafe when used for more than one week or more than five times per year. The product should not be used during pregnancy. It can stimulate contractions in the uterus and may cause premature birth. This product should be avoided during pregnancy.

BREAST-FEEDING: The product may be found in breast milk. This product should not be used when breast-feeding due to its potential to increase melanin production in the infant's skin, which may affect skin color.

COMMON NAME: **Valerian**

PROPER NAME: **Valeriana officinalis**

OTHER NAMES: **Amantilla, baldrian, valeriana, and valeriane**

USES: **To treat insomnia**

FDA PREGNANCY CATEGORY: **None assigned**

VIRTUALLY NO RISK	SLIGHT RISK	MODERATE RISK	STRONG RISK	EXTREME RISK

There is limited evidence that valerian may be effective in treating mild insomnia and improving the quality of sleep. Valerian has not been studied in pregnant women and the potential adverse effects to the fetus are unknown. Women who are pregnant should use caution when taking this product.

BREAST-FEEDING: Valerian is found in breast milk and may cause drowsiness in a breast-fed infant. Caution should be used when breast-feeding.

COMMON NAME: **Yucca**
PROPER NAME: **Yucca schidigera**
OTHER NAMES: **Adam's needle, Joshua tree, soapweed, and Spanish bayonet**
USES: **To treat high blood pressure and high cholesterol**
FDA PREGNANCY CATEGORY: **None assigned**

VIRTUALLY NO RISK	SLIGHT RISK	MODERATE RISK	STRONG RISK	EXTREME RISK

It is not known whether the drug is effective in treating high blood pressure or high cholesterol. Yucca is approved for use in foods and is believed to be safe during pregnancy in the small amounts commonly found in various food products. However, pregnant women should avoid using large amounts of yucca in treating high blood pressure, high cholesterol, or other disorders. When taken in large amounts, the effects on the fetus are unknown.

BREAST-FEEDING: It is not known whether the product is found in breast milk. Caution should be used when breast-feeding.

CHAPTER 5

Vitamin Use During Pregnancy

Vitamin use during pregnancy is often recommended and has become a standard of care. Many physicians want to ensure that their pregnant patients receive all the necessary vitamins and minerals required for the baby to develop as normally and healthily as possible. Some physicians, however, believe that a woman who eats a healthy, well-balanced diet will receive all the vitamins and minerals both she and her baby will need and therefore does not need to take a vitamin supplement.

Most adults do not eat a regular, well-balanced diet on a consistent basis. This may be especially true for the pregnant woman, who may be experiencing some of the stresses of pregnancy, such as morning sickness. Also, our bodies will only store four vitamins (A, D, E, and K) for future use. All other vitamins and minerals must be obtained from the foods we eat on a daily basis or our body goes without them. When certain vitamins are not available, normal development of the fetus could potentially be altered. This reason alone makes a very strong argument for regular use of a good multivitamin during pregnancy. In fact, many physicians are now recommending that women who wish to become pregnant start taking a vitamin supplement three months before they become pregnant. This is why pregnancy is now being referred to as twelve months in duration.

One vitamin that is critical during pregnancy is folic acid. Numerous studies have shown that the lack of folic acid in the mother's diet during the first 16 weeks of pregnancy can lead to neural tube defects (spinal defects) such as spina bifida. At the minimum, a

TABLE 2: VITAMIN REQUIREMENTS DURING PREGNANCY

VITAMINS/MINERALS	NORMAL	DURING PREGNANCY
Vitamin A	2,700IUs	2,700IUs
Vitamin D	200IUs	400IUs
Vitamin E	8mg	10mg
Vitamin K	65mcg	65mcg
Vitamin C	60mg	70mg
Thiamine (B_1)	1.1mg	1.5mg
Riboflavin (B_2)	1.3mg	1.6mg
Niacin	15mg	17mg
Pyridoxine (B_6)	1.6mg	2.2mg
Folic Acid	180mcg	400mcg
Cyanocobalamin (B_{12})	2mcg	2.2mcg
Calcium	800mg	1,200mg
Phosphorus	800mg	1,200mg
Magnesium	280mg	320mg
Iron	15mg	30mg
Zinc	12mg	15mg
Iodine	150mcg	175mcg
Selenium	55mcg	65mcg

IUs = International units
Mcg = micrograms
Mgs = milligrams

pregnant woman should take at least 400 micrograms of folic acid every day and many physicians recommend 1,000 micrograms or 1 milligram per day. All prenatal vitamins contain at least 400 micrograms of folic acid and most contain 1,000 micrograms. Other vitamins, such as iron and calcium, are equally as important to ensure proper development of bones and other major organs in the fetus.

Even though vitamins are very important for the normal growth and development of the fetus, more is not always better. Some women feel the need to supplement their diet with large amounts of various vitamins to ensure proper growth and development of their babies. Most times this is unnecessary, and extremely large doses of some vitamins can actually harm the fetus. This chapter provides information on the potential harm to a fetus when the pregnant mother takes large doses of certain vitamins. Table 2 provides a chart of the recommended dietary allowances for several vitamins and minerals for normal adult women and pregnant women. These recommended allowances come from a joint committee composed of the Food and Nutrition Board, the National Academy of Sciences, and the National Research Council.

FDA pregnancy categories for each vitamin are determined based on large, mega-dosing of these vitamins. Large doses are defined as anything that is more than 2 to 5 times the recommended daily amount required during pregnancy (see Table 2).

VITAMIN: **Vitamin A**
OTHER NAMES: **Retinol**
USE IN THE BODY: **Bone development, reproductive development, and vision**
FDA PREGNANCY CATEGORY: **X (in large doses)**
RISK IN LARGE DOSES:

VIRTUALLY NO RISK	SLIGHT RISK	MODERATE RISK	STRONG RISK	EXTREME RISK

The National Academy of Science recommends that 2,700 IUs of vitamin A should be taken per day. The Food and Drug Administration (FDA) recommends 8,000 IUs of vitamin A per day. Both organizations agree that 8,000 IUs per day is the maximum safe dose during pregnancy. Doses larger than 8,000 IUs have been shown to cause serious birth defects, including cleft palate, heart defects, and various other serious malformations. In fact, the Teratology Society published a position paper in 1987 stating, "Women in their reproductive years should be informed that the excessive use of vitamin A shortly before and during pregnancy could be harmful to their babies." Almost all multivitamins taken during pregnancy contain adequate amounts of vitamin A. Therefore, additional supplementation with vitamin A should be avoided at all costs.

BREAST-FEEDING: Vitamin A is found in breast milk. The potential effects of exposure to excessive amounts of vitamin A to a breast-feeding infant are not known. Women taking large quantities of vitamin A should use extreme caution when breast-feeding.

VITAMIN: **Vitamin B$_1$**
OTHER NAMES: **Thiamine**
USE IN THE BODY: **To ensure proper neurological functioning**
FDA PREGNANCY CATEGORY: **C (in large doses)**
RISK IN LARGE DOSES:

VIRTUALLY NO RISK	SLIGHT RISK	MODERATE RISK	STRONG RISK	EXTREME RISK

When taken in large quantities, the potential effects of thiamine on a fetus are unknown; therefore, large doses of vitamin B$_1$ should not be taken during pregnancy.

BREAST-FEEDING: This vitamin is found in breast milk. However, the American Academy of Pediatrics considers this vitamin to be compatible with breast-feeding. Caution should be used when vitamin B_1 is taken in large quantities.

VITAMIN: **Vitamin B_2**

OTHER NAMES: **Riboflavin**

USE IN THE BODY: **Enzyme production and beneficial biochemical processes**

FDA PREGNANCY CATEGORY: **C (in large doses)**

RISK IN LARGE DOSES:

VIRTUALLY NO RISK	SLIGHT RISK	MODERATE RISK	STRONG RISK	EXTREME RISK
▓	▓	▓		

When taken in large quantities, the potential effects on the fetus are unknown; therefore, large doses of vitamin B_2 should not be taken during pregnancy.

BREAST-FEEDING: This vitamin is found in breast milk. The American Academy of Pediatrics considers this vitamin to be compatible with breast-feeding, but some caution should be used when vitamin B_2 is taken in large quantities.

VITAMIN: **Vitamin B_6**

OTHER NAMES: **Pyridoxine**

USE IN THE BODY: **Metabolism of amino acids and carbohydrates**

FDA PREGNANCY CATEGORY: **C (in large doses)**

RISK IN LARGE DOSES:

VIRTUALLY NO RISK	SLIGHT RISK	MODERATE RISK	STRONG RISK	EXTREME RISK
▓	▓	▓		

Vitamin B_6 is sometimes used to treat nausea and vomiting during pregnancy. There are no clinical studies that prove large doses of vitamin B_6 are effective for this use. In fact, large doses of vitamin B_6 may cause pyridoxine-dependency seizures in a newborn; therefore, it should be used with extreme caution during pregnancy.

BREAST-FEEDING: Very high doses of vitamin B_6 have been shown to inhibit milk production in the mother. In one study, 95 percent of the women taking 600mg of vitamin B_6 per day stopped producing significant amounts of milk. Large doses of vitamin B_6 should not be taken during breast-feeding.

VITAMIN: **Vitamin B_{12}**
OTHER NAMES: **Cyanocobalamin**
USE IN THE BODY: **Cell reproduction and normal growth**
FDA PREGNANCY CATEGORY: **C (in large doses)**
RISK IN LARGE DOSES:

VIRTUALLY NO RISK	SLIGHT RISK	MODERATE RISK	STRONG RISK	EXTREME RISK

There is no data available that documents the effects of taking large doses of vitamin B_{12} during pregnancy; therefore, its effects on the fetus are unknown. Caution should be used when taking extremely high doses (10 to 20 times the normal recommended daily amount) of vitamin B_{12}. However, women who are deficient in vitamin B_{12} may be at a higher risk for birth defects developing in the infant. Any multivitamin taken during pregnancy should contain at least 2.2mcg of vitamin B_{12} to avoid this deficiency.

BREAST-FEEDING: This vitamin is found in breast milk. The American Academy of Pediatrics considers this vitamin to be compatible with breast-feeding, but some caution should be used when vitamin B_{12} is taken in large quantities.

VITAMIN: **Vitamin C**

OTHER NAMES: **Ascorbic acid**

USE IN THE BODY: **Tissue repair and numerous metabolic processes**

FDA PREGNANCY CATEGORY: **C (in large doses)**

RISK IN LARGE DOSES:

VIRTUALLY NO RISK	SLIGHT RISK	MODERATE RISK	STRONG RISK	EXTREME RISK

Excessive doses of vitamin C do not seem to pose a major risk to the fetus. One study found no direct adverse effects on the fetus in mothers who took up to 2,000mg per day of vitamin C. However, the adverse effects of extremely high doses (greater than 2,000mg) on the fetus are not known; therefore, large doses of this vitamin should be used with some caution during pregnancy.

BREAST-FEEDING: This vitamin is found in breast milk. The American Academy of Pediatrics considers this vitamin to be compatible with breast-feeding, but some caution should still be used.

VITAMIN: **Vitamin D**

OTHER NAMES: **Calciferol**

USE IN THE BODY: **Bone development**

FDA PREGNANCY CATEGORY: **D (in large doses)**

RISK IN LARGE DOSES:

VIRTUALLY NO RISK	SLIGHT RISK	MODERATE RISK	STRONG RISK	EXTREME RISK

Large amounts of vitamin D have been shown to cause birth defects in animals. However, there are no studies available in humans regarding the use of high doses of vitamin D during pregnancy. Vitamin D aids calcium absorption and large amounts may cause high levels of calcium in the mother and fetus. In rare cases, this may cause mental retardation and heart deformities; therefore, large doses of Vitamin D should not be taken during pregnancy.

BREAST-FEEDING: This vitamin is found in breast milk. The American Academy of Pediatrics considers this vitamin to be compatible with breast-feeding when taken in normal quantities.

VITAMIN: **Vitamin E**
OTHER NAMES: **Tocopherols**
USE IN THE BODY: **Protects cells from damage**
FDA PREGNANCY CATEGORY: **C (in large doses)**
RISK IN LARGE DOSES:

VIRTUALLY NO RISK	SLIGHT RISK	MODERATE RISK	STRONG RISK	EXTREME RISK

Large doses of vitamin E do not seem to pose a major risk to the fetus. One study found no direct adverse effects on the fetus in mothers who took up to 400 IUs per day of vitamin E starting in weeks 18 to 22. Another group of women took between 600 IUs and 900 IUs during the last two months of pregnancy and no adverse effects were observed in the fetus. However, the adverse effects of extremely high doses on the fetus are not known; therefore, such large doses of vitamin E should be used with caution during pregnancy.

BREAST-FEEDING: This vitamin is found in breast milk. The potential effects of exposure to a breast-feeding infant when the mother takes large doses are not known. Nursing mothers taking large doses of this vitamin should use caution when breast-feeding. Some breast-feeding mothers will apply vitamin E oil to sore nipples. This can significantly increase the blood levels of vitamin E in the infant. The long-term effects of this on the infant are not known; therefore, caution should be used when applying vitamin E to the nipples.

VITAMIN: **Beta-carotene**

OTHER NAMES: **Provitamin A**

USE IN THE BODY: **For several biochemical processes**

FDA PREGNANCY CATEGORY: **C (in large doses)**

RISK IN LARGE DOSES:

VIRTUALLY NO RISK	SLIGHT RISK	MODERATE RISK	STRONG RISK	EXTREME RISK
░░░░░	░░░░░	░░░░░		

When taken in large quantities, beta-carotene's adverse effects on the fetus are unknown; however, high doses are believed to be potentially toxic to the fetus and therefore should not be taken during pregnancy.

BREAST-FEEDING: Beta-carotene is found in breast milk. The potential effects of exposure to excessive amounts of beta-carotene to a breast-feeding infant are not known. Nursing mothers taking large quantities of beta-carotene should use some caution when breast-feeding.

MINERAL: **Iron**

OTHER NAMES: **Ferrous sulfate, Feosol, and ferrous gluconate**

USE IN THE BODY: **For oxygen transport by the red blood cells**

FDA PREGNANCY CATEGORY: **C (in large doses)**

RISK IN LARGE DOSES:

VIRTUALLY NO RISK	SLIGHT RISK	MODERATE RISK	STRONG RISK	EXTREME RISK
░░░░░	░░░░░	░░░░░		

The use of iron supplements during pregnancy is common. The Recommended Daily Allowance (RDA) for iron during pregnancy is 30mg per day. Excessively exceeding the RDA is not recommended due to potential harm to the fetus. Consult your physician to determine the correct dosage of any vitamin or mineral supplement during pregnancy.

BREAST-FEEDING: Iron is found in breast milk. The potential effects of exposure to large quantities of this supplement on a breast-feeding infant are not known. Nursing mothers taking large amounts of iron supplement should use caution when breast-feeding.

VITAMIN: **Niacin**
OTHER NAMES: **Niacinamide and vitamin B₃**
USE IN THE BODY: **For glucose utilization and other biochemical processes**
FDA PREGNANCY CATEGORY: **C (in large doses)**
RISK IN LARGE DOSES:

VIRTUALLY NO RISK	SLIGHT RISK	MODERATE RISK	STRONG RISK	EXTREME RISK

When taken in large quantities, the potential effects of niacin on the fetus are unknown; therefore, large doses should not be used during pregnancy.

BREAST-FEEDING: This vitamin is found in breast milk. The American Academy of Pediatrics considers it to be compatible with breast-feeding, but caution should be used when niacin is taken in large quantities.

VITAMIN: **Pantothenic acid**
OTHER NAMES: **Vitamin B₅**
USE IN THE BODY: **Production of several proteins, carbohydrates, and hormones**
FDA PREGNANCY CATEGORY: **C (in large doses)**
RISK IN LARGE DOSES:

VIRTUALLY NO RISK	SLIGHT RISK	MODERATE RISK	STRONG RISK	EXTREME RISK

When taken in large quantities, the potential effects of pantothenic acid on the fetus are unknown; therefore, large doses should not be taken during pregnancy.

BREAST-FEEDING: This vitamin is found in breast milk. The American Academy of Pediatrics considers this vitamin to be compatible with breast-feeding, but caution should be used when pantothenic acid is taken in large quantities.

CHAPTER 6

Household Products, Chemicals, and Toxins

Many women think that all household products, appliances, and chemicals have been tested and proven safe for use during pregnancy when in fact many have not. There is a common misconception that just because a product is safe for consumer use then it must be safe to use during pregnancy. In fact, most products and household chemicals have not been tested as to their effects on the fetus. Conversely, misinformation abounds that many household products and chemicals are potentially harmful during pregnancy. The outcome is that most pregnant women do not know what to believe when it comes to what is potentially harmful to the unborn child and what is not. This chapter discusses the potential harm from some of the most common household products and chemicals and seeks to clear up a lot of the confusion and misinformation. The key thing to remember about household chemicals and products is to minimize exposure whenever possible and to use them in moderation. Problems are most likely to occur as a result of overexposure or prolonged use over long periods of time.

PRODUCT: **Alcohol**

OTHER NAMES: **Beer, wine, hard liquor, spirits, etc.**

GENERIC NAME: **Ethanol**

FDA PREGNANCY CATEGORY: **D (X in large quantities or for prolonged periods)**

VIRTUALLY NO RISK	SLIGHT RISK	MODERATE RISK	STRONG RISK	EXTREME RISK

Alcohol is known to cause birth defects, especially when the mother drinks during the first two months of pregnancy. Even moderate drinking has been associated with an increased risk of miscarriage and developmental and behavioral problems in infants. Heavy drinking is related to a whole host of birth defects that is collectively termed fetal alcohol syndrome (FAS). Fetal alcohol syndrome can include not only severe birth defects but developmental and behavioral disorders in the infant after birth as well. Mild FAS and low birth weight have been seen in infants whose mothers consumed as little as two drinks per day in early pregnancy. Full-blown FAS is usually seen when pregnant women consume four or more drinks per day over the course of the pregnancy. The American Council on Science and Health recommends that pregnant women consume not more than two drinks daily on an occasional basis. However, the safest recommendation for women who are pregnant or who are planning to become pregnant is to avoid alcohol completely.

BREAST-FEEDING: Alcohol is found in breast milk. The potential effects of exposure to alcohol on a breast-feeding infant are not completely understood. Women drinking large amounts of alcohol should use caution when breast-feeding.

PRODUCT: **Bug Sprays and Pesticides**

FDA PREGNANCY CATEGORY: **None assigned**

VIRTUALLY NO RISK	SLIGHT RISK	MODERATE RISK	STRONG RISK	EXTREME RISK

Most exposure to bug sprays is accidental and in very small amounts. Many pregnant women worry when they have been in area where bug sprays and pesticides have been used and they can smell them. There are no known documented cases of birth defects due to this type of exposure to bug sprays; therefore, such short exposure should not cause any problems. However, long-term exposure may cause serious birth defects in the fetus. Pesticides applied to lawns and gardens should not cause a significant risk to the fetus if exposure is from casual contact. However, pregnant women should avoid spreading or applying pesticides and chemicals to lawns and gardens themselves because the exact risk to the fetus is still unknown.

BREAST-FEEDING: It is not known to what extent these products are found in breast milk. Women who breast-feed should avoid long-term exposure to these types of chemicals.

PRODUCT: **Caffeine**

FDA PREGNANCY CATEGORY: **B**

VIRTUALLY NO RISK	SLIGHT RISK	MODERATE RISK	STRONG RISK	EXTREME RISK

Caffeine is one of the most popular drugs in the world. In fact, two cups of coffee can contain as much as 450mg of caffeine, compared to soft drinks and herbal teas, which have about 47mg. Consumption of moderate amounts of caffeine does not appear to affect the fetus. However, high doses of caffeine, four to six cups of coffee, have been associated with an increased risk of miscarriage and low birth weight. When high doses of caffeine are combined with cigarette smoking, the risk of delivering a baby with lower birth weight is significantly greater. Therefore, women should drink caffeinated beverages in moderation during pregnancy—no more than two cups of coffee should be consumed per day. Since soft drinks and herbals teas contain significantly less caffeine than coffee, consumption of these products should be limited to two to six servings per day. However, beverages that do not contain caffeine are always preferred.

BREAST-FEEDING: This product is found in breast milk. The American Academy of Pediatrics considers caffeine use to be compatible with breast-feeding, but some caution should still be taken. Nursing mothers who drink large amounts of caffeinated beverages may notice irritability and poor sleeping habits in infants who breast-feed.

TOXIN: **Carbon Monoxide**

FDA PREGNANCY CATEGORY: **None assigned**

VIRTUALLY NO RISK	SLIGHT RISK	MODERATE RISK	STRONG RISK	EXTREME RISK

Carbon monoxide is known to cause birth defects in the fetus. One of the most common problems is central nervous system defects and disorders. Pregnant women exposed to a leaking or malfunctioning gas furnace should contact their physician immediately to determine the potential adverse effect on the fetus.

BREAST-FEEDING: It is not known whether or how much carbon monoxide is found in breast milk after exposure. Women should use caution when breast-feeding, especially shortly after exposure.

AGENT: **Electric Shock**

FDA PREGNANCY CATEGORY: **D**

VIRTUALLY NO RISK	SLIGHT RISK	MODERATE RISK	STRONG RISK	EXTREME RISK

There are published reports of five different types of electrical shock or exposure during pregnancy: accidental electric shock in the home, lightning strikes, electroconvulsive therapy, electric shock in cardiac arrest/irregular heartbeat, and from a stun gun (Taser weapon). An electrical shock sustained in the home can cause a variety of effects on the fetus, depending on the source and strength of the shock. A mild electrical shock should have a minimal effect on the fetus. However, a moderate electrical shock has caused miscarriage and major malformations in the fetus. Pregnant women who experience any type of household electrical shock, even if deemed minor, should contact their physician. Lightning strikes to humans are often fatal. Pregnant women who survive a lightning strike can expect about a 50 percent chance of survival of the fetus. Some forms of electroconvulsive therapy are considered safe during pregnancy, but other forms of treatment should be considered instead. Electrical shock administered during cardiac arrest/irregular heartbeat is considered a safe procedure during pregnancy; in fact, it may be required to save the life of the mother and child. Exposure to a stun gun or Taser device has been shown to cause miscarriage. The closer the electrical current from one of these weapons is applied to the uterus, the more likely it is that miscarriage will occur.

BREAST-FEEDING: It is not known how direct electrical shock affects breast milk or breast-feeding. Some caution should be used when breast-feeding shortly after electrical shock.

PRODUCT: **Hair Bleach**

FDA PREGNANCY CATEGORY: **None assigned**

VIRTUALLY NO RISK	SLIGHT RISK	MODERATE RISK	STRONG RISK	EXTREME RISK
▓▓▓▓▓▓	▓▓▓▓▓▓			

Most hair bleaching formulas contain hydrogen peroxide, which is changed to water and oxygen rapidly when exposed to air. In general, most exposures to hair bleach are at low levels and do not cause adverse effects to the fetus. Currently, there are no well-documented reports of adverse effects in either animals or humans and this product is considered safe to use topically during pregnancy. However, if the patient experiences signs and symptoms of toxic effects, she should contact her physician immediately.

BREAST-FEEDING: These chemicals should not be found in breast milk. Nursing mothers may breast-feed after using these products.

PRODUCT: **Hair Dyes and Coloring Agents**

FDA PREGNANCY CATEGORY: **None assigned**

VIRTUALLY NO RISK	SLIGHT RISK	MODERATE RISK	STRONG RISK	EXTREME RISK
▓▓▓▓▓▓	▓▓▓▓▓▓			

The effects of topically applied hair dyes and coloring agents have been studied in rabbits, and no systemic or adverse effects have been found. These products were also tested on pregnant rats and no biologically significant soft tissue or skeletal problems were found in the fetuses. These products have not been tested in humans and the chance for serious adverse effects to the fetus appears to be slight.

BREAST-FEEDING: These chemicals do not pass into breast milk; therefore, nursing mothers may breast-feed after using these products.

BRAND NAME: **Iodine (topical)**

OTHER NAMES: **Betadine, iodide, and povidone iodine**

GENERIC NAME: **Iodine**

FDA PREGNANCY CATEGORY: **D**

VIRTUALLY NO RISK	SLIGHT RISK	MODERATE RISK	STRONG RISK	EXTREME RISK

Dietary iodine is necessary for proper thyroid function and is not harmful to the fetus when consumed as part of a well-balanced diet. However, clinical studies have shown potentially hazardous effects on the fetus when iodine was used topically by the mother on a cut or wound. Vaginal douches that contain iodine should be avoided as well. These products may cause thyroid and heart problems in the fetus, which can be fatal. Many over-the-counter products contain iodine or iodide and should be avoided at all costs.

BREAST-FEEDING: This drug is found in breast milk. The potential effects of exposure to this drug on a breast-feeding infant are not known. Nursing mothers taking large amounts of iodine should use extreme caution when breast-feeding.

PRODUCT: **Microwave Ovens**

FDA PREGNANCY CATEGORY: **None assigned**

VIRTUALLY NO RISK	SLIGHT RISK	MODERATE RISK	STRONG RISK	EXTREME RISK

There is no way to receive exposure from a microwave oven without bypassing or breaking several safety locks. Theoretically if there were a leak, exposure could potentially lead to the development of birth defects. However, as long as the woman stayed several feet away from an operating microwave, exposure through a leak would be minimal. Microwave ovens, when used properly, are considered safe during pregnancy.

BREAST-FEEDING: These devices do not affect milk production or pose any risk to a breast-feeding infant unless the microwaves are directed specifically to the breast area.

PRODUCT: **Nicotine (from cigarettes)**
FDA PREGNANCY CATEGORY: **D**

VIRTUALLY NO RISK	SLIGHT RISK	MODERATE RISK	STRONG RISK	EXTREME RISK
▓	▓	▓	▓	

Smoking has been shown to be harmful to the fetus. Nicotine, a chemical ingested during smoking, has been shown to affect fetal breathing due to a decrease in blood flow. Miscarriage has also been reported when nicotine is used during pregnancy. Therefore, mothers who continue to smoke during pregnancy have a significantly higher risk of having a baby with some sort of birth defect or major malformation.

BREAST-FEEDING: Components of cigarette smoke are found in breast milk. The potential effects of exposure to these components on a breast-feeding infant are not known. Nursing mothers who smoke should use some caution when breast-feeding.

BRAND NAME: **NutraSweet**
OTHER NAMES: **Equal**
GENERIC NAME: **aspartame**
FDA PREGNANCY CATEGORY: **B**

VIRTUALLY NO RISK	SLIGHT RISK	MODERATE RISK	STRONG RISK	EXTREME RISK
▓	▓			

NutraSweet is probably the most extensively studied food additive ever approved by the Food and Drug Administration. It is approximately 200 times sweeter than sugar. Drinks and foods flavored with NutraSweet are considered safe for consumption in moderation during pregnancy and have no effect on the fetus. However, women with phenylketonuria (PKU), a birth defect in which protein metabolism is inhibited and causes the amino acid phenylalanine to accumulate in the blood, should use caution. NutraSweet contains phenylalanine. In women with PKU, excessive phenylalanine in the bloodstream of the mother can be toxic to the fetus.

BREAST-FEEDING: This product is found in breast milk. The American Academy of Pediatrics considers this additive to be compatible with breast-feeding, but caution should be used in women or infants with phenylketonuria (PKU).

PRODUCT: **Organic Solvents (benzene, acetone, fingernail polish remover, some cleaning agents, etc.)**
FDA PREGNANCY CATEGORY: **None assigned**

VIRTUALLY NO RISK	SLIGHT RISK	MODERATE RISK	STRONG RISK	EXTREME RISK

Exposure to organic solvents around the house in small quantities and for very short periods of time is usually considered not to be a problem during pregnancy, but the true effects of this exposure are still unknown. However, exposure to industrial organic solvents for longer periods of time at work could pose a very serious problem. Exposure to industrial solvents has been shown to cause liver problems, heart defects, blood abnormalities, and other serious birth defects in the fetus; therefore, extreme caution should be used when exposed to these products during pregnancy.

BREAST-FEEDING: It is not known whether these chemicals are found in breast milk. Nursing mothers should use some caution when breast-feeding.

PRODUCT: **Paint (house)**

FDA PREGNANCY CATEGORY: **None assigned**

VIRTUALLY NO RISK	SLIGHT RISK	MODERATE RISK	STRONG RISK	EXTREME RISK

Many pregnant women will paint one or more rooms of their house in anticipation of the arrival of their new child. Water-based paints and latex paints are definitely safer choices than oil-based paints and pose less risk to the fetus. Water-based paints usually do not have volatile vapors that may be toxic to the mother and fetus. Exposure to oil-based paints is believed to be safe as well when exposure to the fumes is for very short periods of time and in well-ventilated areas. Pregnant women should avoid paints that contain lead. Most commercially available paints do not contain lead, but some glass-staining materials do. Pregnant women should also avoid scraping walls that were painted with lead-based paints. Exposure to lead can cause skeletal defects, central nervous system abnormalities, and even death of the fetus. Pregnant women who want to paint should use water-based or latex products to minimize potential risk to the fetus.

BREAST-FEEDING: It is not known whether the chemicals from paint are found in breast milk. Nursing mothers should use some caution when breast-feeding.

PRODUCT: **Permanent Solutions for Hair (Perms)**

FDA PREGNANCY CATEGORY: **None assigned**

VIRTUALLY NO RISK	SLIGHT RISK	MODERATE RISK	STRONG RISK	EXTREME RISK

Many women use permanent solutions to give their hair a curly or wavy appearance. Permanent kits contain two solutions, a waving solution and a neutralizing solution. The waving solution may cause some local irritation, but no adverse effects have been seen when used on animals that are pregnant. The neutralizing solution is composed mainly of hydrogen peroxide, which is changed to water and oxygen rapidly when exposed to air and does not cause adverse effects in the fetus. Therefore, permanent solutions are generally considered safe for use by pregnant women.

BREAST-FEEDING: These chemicals should not be found in breast milk. Nursing mothers may breast-feed after using these products.

PRODUCT: **Silicon Breast Implants**
FDA PREGNANCY CATEGORY: **C**

VIRTUALLY NO RISK	SLIGHT RISK	MODERATE RISK	STRONG RISK	EXTREME RISK

Silicon breast implants are composed of a shell made of polydimethylsiloxane gum (PDMS) filled with either saline, silicone oil, or PDMS gel. The prevalence of rupture of these implants is believed to be 4 to 6 percent. More than two million women have received silicone implants in the U.S. Several serious health concerns have been raised regarding the adverse effects when implants rupture or leak. When this happens, the body may perceive these compounds as foreign and elicit an immune response. The same response may be seen in the fetus. However, the clinical significance of this immune response is not known and many physicians feel it is insignificant. Women with breast implants should, however, contact their doctor immediately if they suspect there is a problem.

BREAST-FEEDING: This product is found in breast milk if leaking or rupture has occurred and may be harmful to a breast-feeding infant; therefore, extreme caution should be exercised by nursing mothers.

BRAND NAME: **Sweet 'N Low Sweetener**

OTHER NAMES: **Artificial sweetener**

GENERIC NAME: **saccharin**

FDA PREGNANCY CATEGORY: **C**

VIRTUALLY NO RISK	SLIGHT RISK	MODERATE RISK	STRONG RISK	EXTREME RISK

Saccharin is a sugar substitute that is typically found in pink packets at most restaurants. It is approximately 300 times sweeter than sugar. Years ago saccharin, in high doses, was found to cause cancer in lab mice. Saccharin was never found to cause cancer in humans; however, the final verdict is still out. Therefore, it is recommended that saccharin should not be used by pregnant women. A better sugar substitute is aspartame (NutraSweet or Equal), which is a safer alternative for most women. The best alternative, however, is to stick with plain sugar, unless diabetic. After all, one sugar packet contains less than 20 calories. For most women, the risk of using saccharin while pregnant does not justify the benefit of saving 20 calories.

BREAST-FEEDING: This product is found in breast milk. The potential effects of exposure to this drug on a breast-feeding infant are not known and the chances of harm to the infant are small. However, women ingesting large amounts of saccharin should use some caution when breast-feeding.

PRODUCT: **Video Display Terminals and Computer Monitors**

FDA PREGNANCY CATEGORY: **None assigned**

VIRTUALLY NO RISK	SLIGHT RISK	MODERATE RISK	STRONG RISK	EXTREME RISK

Several years ago some scientists suspected that video display terminals and computer monitors had adverse effects on the fetus after several miscarriages were reported. However, scientific research has confirmed that that these devices do not emit X rays, microwaves, or other radiation at levels that would be harmful to either the mother or the fetus. Current data indicates that these devices do not increase the risk of birth defects in the fetus.

BREAST-FEEDING: These devices do not affect milk production or pose any risk to a breast-feeding infant.

PROCEDURE: **X ray**

FDA PREGNANCY CATEGORY: **None assigned**

VIRTUALLY NO RISK	SLIGHT RISK	MODERATE RISK	STRONG RISK	EXTREME RISK

Exposure to the radiation from X rays in doses less than 5 rads is not associated with an increase in the incidence of birth defects. In the dosage range of 5 to 15 rads, there may be an increased risk of birth defects. For dosages of more than 15 rads, there appears to be a two to three times greater risk of birth defects in the fetus. The normal exposure range for diagnostic X rays, including dental X rays, generally should be far below a level that would cause birth defects. However, the radiologist involved should be told that the patient is pregnant and assess the potential risk to the mother and fetus.

BREAST-FEEDING: These devices do not affect milk production or pose any risk to a breast-feeding infant unless the X rays are directed specifically to the breast area.

Appendix
Other Sources of Information

Women who would like to receive more information regarding the potential risks of drugs, chemicals, or toxins to the fetus can contact one of the following sources as well:

1. **MOTHERISK PROGRAM.** Tel. (416) 813-6780 or www.motherisk.org

2. **ORGANIZATION OF TERATOLOGY INFORMATION SERVICE.** Tel. (801) 328-2229 or http://orpheus.ucsd.edu/ctis/

3. **CALIFORNIA TERATOGEN INFORMATION SERVICE.** Tel. (619) 542-2131

4. **FLORIDA TERATOGEN INFORMATION SERVICE.** Tel. (352) 392-3050

5. **ILLINOIS TERATOGEN INFORMATION SERVICE.** Tel. (312) 908-7441

6. **MASSACHUSETTS TERATOGEN INFORMATION SERVICE.** Tel. (781) 466-8474

7. **TEXAS TERATOGEN INFORMATION SERVICE.**

   Tel. (800) 733-4727

8. **UTAH PREGNANCY RISKLINE.**

   Tel. (801) 328-2229

9. **VERMONT PREGNANCY RISK INFORMATION.**

   Tel. (802) 658-4310

Index

B

Baby, development of, 3–6
Bacitracin, neomycin, polymyxin B and (Neosporin), 161
Backache, treating, 148–149
Bacterial eye infections, treating, 114
Bacterial infections, treating, 24–25, 27–28, 32–33, 34–35, 36, 46, 50, 53–54, 55–56, 65, 74, 80–81, 110–111, 121, 122, 127
Bacterial skin infections, treating, 25–26
Bacterial vaginal infections, treating, 79
Bactrim DS (sulfamethoxazole and trimethoprim), 24–25
Bactroban (mupirocin), 25–26
Bayberry, 186
Bayer Aspirin (aspirin), 138
Beclomethasone dipropionate (Beclovent), 26
Beclomethasone dipropionate (Vancenase AQ DS), 120
Beclovent (beclomethasone dipropionate), 26
Bedwetting, treating, 114–115
Bee pollen, 186
Behavioral problems, treating, 59
Benadryl (diphenhydramine), 19, 139
Benazepril (Lotensin), see Accupril
Benazepril, amiodipine and (Lotrel), 75
Bentyl (dicyclomine), 27
Benzocaine (Solarcaine), 171–172
Benzodiazepine family, 21
Benzoic acid, methenamine, phenyl salicyclate, methylene blue, atropine, hyoscyamine and (Urised), 118–119
Benzonatate (Tessalon), 112
Benzoyl peroxide 10% (Oxy–10), 166
Beta-blockers, 63, 73
Beta-carotene, 217
Betamethasone dipropionate, clotrimazole and (Lotrisone), 76
Biaxin (clarithromycin), 27–28
Bilberry, 187

Bipolar disorder, treating, 70–71
Birth control pills, see Oral contraceptives
Birth defects, chances of, 6–7
Bisacodyl (Correctol), 146
Bisacodyl (Dulcolax), see Correctol
Bismuth subsalicylate (Pepto-Bismol), 167
Bisoprolol and hydrochlorothiazide (Ziac), 126–127
Black Horehound and Ballota, 187–188
Bleeding in newborn after delivery, 45
Blood vessels, fetal, 5
Bluish-colored baby, 65
Bones, fetal, 5
Bonine (meclizine), 139–140
Bowel problems, treating, 190
Brain, fetal, 5
Breast cancer, treating, 86
Breast-feeding
    drugs and, 9–12
    pregnancy and, 1–12
    tips when taking medication while, 10–11
Breast-feeding problems, treating, 188
Breast milk, 9–10
    Beta-carotene in, 217
    Cyanocobalamin (B_{12}) in, 214
    expressing or pumping, 11
    Iron in, 217–218
    Niacin in, 218
    Pantothenic acid (B_5) in, 218–219
    Pyridoxine (B_6) in, 213–214
    Thiamine (B_1) in, 212–213
    Vitamin A in, 211–212
    Vitamin C in, 215
    Vitamin D in, 215–216
    Vitamin E in, 216
Breasts
    enlarged, 1
    tender, 1
Breathing disorders, treating, 14, 99, 106–107, 108–109, 130
Breathing movements, fetal, 6

Ecotrin (enteric-coated aspirin), *see*
    Bayer Aspirin
Ectopic pregnancy, 2
Eczema, treating, 193
Effexor (venlafaxine), 48
Egg, mother's, fertilization of, by
    sperm, 3–4
Egg implantation, problems with, 35
Elasticity of pelvis, 4
Elavil (amitriptyline), 49
Electric shock, 225
Electroconvulsive therapy, 225
ELISA (enzyme-linked immunosor-
    bent assay) techniques, 1
Elocon (mometasone), 49
Embryo, 4, 5
Emetrol (dextrose and fructose), 151
Emphysema, treating, 21, 99, 108–109
Enalapril (Vasotec), 121
Endometrium, 4, 5
Enlarged breasts, 1
Enteric-coated aspirin (Ecotrin), *see*
    Bayer Aspirin
Entex (phenylephrine,
    pseudoephedrine, and
    guaifenesin), 50–51
Enzyme-linked immunosorbent assay
    (ELISA) techniques, 1
Epilepsy, treating, 65–66, 84–85
Epileptic seizures, treating, 45
Epinephrine (Primatene Mist
    Inhaler), 169–170
Ery-Tab (erythromycin base), *see*
    E-Mycin
Erythromycin (E-Mycin), 50
Erythromycin (PCE), *see* E-Mycin
Erythromycin base (Ery-Tab), *see*
    E-Mycin
Esgic (acetaminophen, butalbital, and
    caffeine), *see* Floricet
Estazolam (ProSom), 98
Estrogen, 4
Ethinyl estradiol
    desogestrel and (Ortho-Cept), *see*
        Alesse-28
    levonorgestrel and (Alesse-28),
        16–17

levonorgestrel and (Tri-Levlen), *see*
    Alesse-28
levonorgestrel and (Triphasil), *see*
    Alesse-28
norethindrone and (Loestrin
    Fe 1.5/30), *see* Alesse-28
norethindrone and (Ortho-Novum
    7/7/7), *see* Alesse-28
norgestimate and (Ortho Tri-
    Cyclen), *see* Alesse-28
norgestimate and (Ortho-Cyclen),
    see Alesse-28
norgestrel and (Lo/Orral), *see*
    Alesse-28
Etodolac (Lodine), 71
Evening Primrose, 193
Ex-Lax (senna), 152
Excedrin Extra Strength and Excedrin
    Migraine (acetaminophen,
    aspirin, and caffeine), 152–153
Expectorants in pregnancy, 60
Expressing breast milk, 11
Eyes, fetal, 5

F

Fallopian tubes, 4
False negative results, 2
False positive results, 2
Famotidine (Mylanta AR), *see* Pepcid
    AC
Famotidine (Pepcid AC), 166
Famotidine (Pepcid), 90
FAS (fetal alcohol syndrome), 222
Fast heartbeat, treating, 67–68
Fatty acids, 9
FDA, *see* Food and Drug Administra-
    tion
Feeling of fullness in stomach,
    treating, 191–192
Felodipine (Plendil), 93
Femstat-3 (butaconazole), 153–154
Fertilization of mother's egg by
    sperm, 3–4
Fetal alcohol syndrome (FAS), 222
Fetal distress during labor, 42
Fetal risk from drugs, FDA classifica-
    tion categories of, xv, 8–9

H

Habitrol (nicotine transdermal patch), 58–59
Hair Bleach, 226
Hair Dyes and Coloring Agents, 226
Haldol (haloperidol), 59
Haloperidol (Haldol), 59
Hangover symptoms, treating, 196–197
Hay fever, treating, 186
HCG, *see* Human chorionic gonadotropin
Head lice, treating, 163
Headaches
    migraine, treating, 42–43
    tension, *see* Tension headaches
    treating, 138, 152–153
Heart, fetal, 5
Heart attack, treating, 73
Heart failure, treating, 14–15, 18, 97, 121, 125–126
Heartbeat, fetal, 6
Heartburn, treating, 136, 137–138, 155–156, 158–159, 166, 167, 168, 173, 176, 182, 199–200
Hemorrhoids, treating, 137, 169, 187
Herbal and homeopathic products, 183–207
Herpes cold sores, treating, 129
High blood pressure, treating, 14–15, 16, 18, 28–30, 31–32, 39–40, 47–48, 61–62, 63, 73, 75, 76–77, 87, 93, 97–98, 121, 125–127, 194–195, 207
High cholesterol, treating, 70, 80, 194–195, 207
HIV virus, 10
Home pregnancy kits, 1–2
    tips for using, 2–3
Homeopathic and herbal products, 183–207
Household products in pregnancy, 221–233
Human chorionic gonadotropin (HCG), 4–5
    detecting presence of, 1
    levels of, 2
Human milk, *see* Breast milk

Humibid LA (guaifenesin), 60
Humilin N (insulin), 60–61
Hydrochlorothiazide
    bisoprolol and (Ziac), 126–127
    lisinopril and (Zestoretic), 125–126
    losartan and (Hyzaar), 61–62
    triamterene and (Dyazide), 47
    triamterene and (Maxzide), *see* Dyazide
Hydrocodone
    acetaminophen and (Lortab), 74–75
    acetaminophen and (Vicodin), 122–123
Hydrocortisone (Cortaid), 147
Hydrogen peroxide, 226
Hyoscyamine (Levsin), 69
Hyoscyamine, methenamine, phenyl salicyclate, methylene blue, benzoic acid, atropine and (Urised), 118–119
Hypertension, treating, 22–23
Hypochondria, treating, 187–188
Hypospadias, 28
Hysteria, treating, 187–188
Hytrin (terazosin), 61
Hyzaar (losartan and hydrochlorothiazide), 61–62

I

Ibuprofen (Advil), 134–135
Ibuprofen (Motrin), 81–82
Ibuprofen (Motrin IB), *see* Advil
Ibuprofen (Nuprin), *see* Advil
Imipramine (Tofranil), 114–115
Imitrex (sumatriptan), 62–63
Immune system, infant's, 10
Immune system problems, treating, 94–95
Imodium AD (loperamide), 157
Impetigo, treating, 25–26
Improving memory, 196
Indapamide (Lozol), 76–77
Inderal (propranolol), 63
Infant's immune system, 10
Infection, preventing, 161
Infections, treating, 19–20
Infertility, 51

Lorazepam (Ativan), 20–21
Lortab (acetaminophen and
    hydrocodone), 74–75
Losartan (Cozaar), 39–40
Losartan and hydrochlorothiazide
    (Hyzaar), 61–62
Loss of appetite, treating, 191–192
Lotensin (benazepril), *see* Accupril
Lotrel (amiodipine and benazepril), 75
Lotrimin AF (clotrimazole), 158
Lotrisone (clotrimazole and betametha-
    sone dipropionate), 76
Lovastatin (Mevacor), 80
Lozol (indapamide), 76–77
Lung development problems, 40
Lung inflammation, treating, 24, 26
Luvox (fluvoxamine), 77

M

Maalox (magnesium hydroxide and
    aluminum hydroxide), 158–159
Macrobid (nitrofurantoin), 77–78
Macrodantin (nitrofurantoin), *see*
    Macrobid
Macrophages, 9
Magnesium, 210
Magnesium hydroxide (Phillip's Milk
    of Magnesia), 168
Magnesium hydroxide and aluminum
    hydroxide (Maalox), 158–159
Magnesium salicylate (Doan's Pills),
    148–149
Magnesium trisilicate, aluminum
    hydroxide, alginic acid and
    (Gaviscon), 155–156
Maintaining flow of breast milk, 11
Mania, treating, 42–43
Manic episodes, treating, 70–71
Masculinization, 17
Maxzide (triamterene and
    hydrochlorothiazide), *see*
    Dyazide
Meclizine (Bonine), 139–140
Medical literature, 13
Melatonin, 201
Menstrual cramps, treating,
    152–153, 192

Menstrual pain, treating, 81–82,
    123–124
Mental development disorders, 7
Meridia (silbutramine), 78–79
Mesalamine (Asacol), 20
Mesalamine (Pentasa), 89–90
Metamucil (psyllium), *see* Citrucel
Metaxalone (Skelaxin), 108
Metformin (Glucophage), 57
Methenamine, phenyl salicyclate,
    methylene blue, benzoic acid,
    atropine, hyoscyamine and
    (Urised), 118–119
Methylcellulose (Citrucel), 143
Methyldopa (Aldomet), 16
Methylene blue, methenamine,
    phenyl salicyclate, benzoic
    acid, atropine, hyoscyamine
    and (Urised), 118–119
Methylphenidate (Ritalin), 105
Metoclopramide (Reglan), 101
Metoprolol (Toprol XL), *see* Lopressor
MetroGel Vaginal (metronidazole), 79
Metronidazole (Flagyl), 53–54
Metronidazole (MetroGel Vaginal), 79
Metroprolol tartrate (Lopressor), 73
Mevacor (lovastatin), 80
Miconazole (Monistat 7), 159
Micronase (glyburide), *see* DiaBeta
Micronized glyburide (Glynase), *see*
    DiaBeta
Microwave Ovens, 227
Migraine headaches, treating, 42–43,
    62–63, 194
Milk, breast, *see* Breast milk
Milk Thistle, 202
Minocin (minocycline), 80–81
Minocycline (Minocin), 80–81
Mirtazapine (Remeron), 102
Mometasone (Elocon), 49
Mometasone furoate (Nasonex), 83–84
Monistat 7 (miconazole), 159
Monoclonal antibodies, 1
Monopril (fosinopril), *see* Accupril
Morning sickness, 1
    treating, 189, 195
Morning urine samples, 2

Simvastatin (Zocor), *see* Mevacor
Sine-Aid (acetaminophen and pseudo-
    ephedrine), *see* Tylenol Sinus
Sinus infection, xiv
Sinusitis, treating, 147–148
Sinutab (acetaminophen, chlorpheni-
    ramine, and pseudoephedrine),
    see Theraflu
Sio-bid (theophylline), 108–109
Skelaxin (metaxalone), 108
Skin disorders, treating, 193
Skin irritations, treating, 140–141,
    147
Skin rashes, treating, 49
Sleep aids, 180
Smoking, quitting, 58–59, 161–162
Sneezing, treating, 139
Sodium, docusate, prenatal vitamin
    with (Prenate Ultra), 95
Sodium bicarbonate and potassium
    bicarbonate (Alka-Seltzer), 136
Sodium biphosphate (Fleet Enema),
    154–155
Solarcaine (benzocaine), 171–172
Soma (carisoprodol), 109
Sominex (diphenhydramine), *see*
    Benadryl
Sore throat, treating, 142, 177–178
Sour stomach, treating, 137–138,
    158–159, 166, 168, 173, 176
Sperm, fertilization of mother's egg
    by, 3–4
Spinal cord, fetal, 5
Spontaneous abortions, 4
Sporanox (itraconazole), 110
St. John's-wort, 203–204
Stages of pregnancy, 5
Stillbirths, xiii
Stomach cramps, treating, 167
Stomach disorders, treating, 27
Stomach problems, treating, 190
Stomach spasms, treating, 69
Stomach ulcers, treating, 23–24, 90,
    125
Stomachache, treating, 194
Stool softeners, 144–145
Stress, treating, 200

Stun gun, 225
Sucking movements, fetal, 6
Sucralfate (Carafate), 30
Sudafed (pseudoephedrine), 172
Sulfamethoxazole and trimethoprim
    (Bactrim DS), 24–25
Sulindac (Clinoril), 38
Sumatriptan (Imitrex), 62–63
Sumycin (tetracycline), *see* Minocin
Sunburn, treating, 171–172
Suprax (cefixime), 110–111
Surfak (docusate calcium), *see* Colace
Sweet 'N Low Sweetener, 232
Swelling, treating, 49
Symptoms of pregnancy, 1
Synthroid (levothyroxine), 111

T
Tagamet HB (cimetidine), 173
Tamoxifen (Nolvadex), 86
Taser weapon, 225
Tavist-D (clemastine and
    pseudoephedrine), 174
Temazepam (Restoril), 102–103
Tender breasts, 1
Tenormin (atenolol), *see* Lopressor
Tension headaches, xiii
    treating, 51–53, 92–93
Terazosin (Hytrin), 61
Terbinafine (Lamisil), 67
Tessalon (benzonatate), 112
Tetracycline, xiv
Tetracycline (Sumycin), *see* Minocin
Theo-Dur (theophylline anhydrous),
    see Sio-bid
Theophylline (Sio-bid), 108–109
Theophylline anhydrous (Theo-Dur),
    see Sio-bid
Theraflu (acetaminophen,
    pseudoephedrine, and chlor-
    pheniramine), 175
Thiamine (B$_1$), 210, 212–213
Thromboembolic disorders, treating,
    39
Thyroid hormone replacement
    therapy, 68–69, 111
Tiagabine (Gabitril), 56

Tigan (trimethobenzamide), 112–113
Tightness of chest, treating, 169–170
Tilade (nedocromil), 113
Tinactin (tolnaftate), 176
Tioconazole (Vagistat-1), 181
Tobradex (tobramycin and dexamethasone), 114
Tobramycin and dexamethasone (Tobradex), 114
Tocopherols, 199
Toenail fungus, treating, 67
Tofranil (imipramine), 114–115
Tolnaftate (Tinactin), 176
Topical pain relief, 171–172
Topically applied creams, ointments, and nasal sprays, 11
Toprol XL (metoprolol), see Lopressor
Toxins in pregnancy, 221–233
Tramadol (Ultram), 118
Transdermal patch, nicotine (Habitrol), 58–59
Tranxene (clorazepate), 115
Trazodone (Desyrel), 43
Tretinoin (Retin-A), 103
Tri-Levlen (levonorgestrel and ethinyl estradiol), see Alesse-28
Triamcinolone (Azmacort), 24
Triamcinolone acetonide (Nasacort), 83
Triamterene
  and hydrochlorothiazide (Dyazide), 47
  and hydrochlorothiazide (Maxzide), see Dyazide
Trichomoniasis, treating, 53–54
Trimesters, 5
Trimethobenzamide (Tigan), 112–113
Trimethoprim, sulfamethoxazole and (Bactrim DS), 24–25
Trimox (amoxicillin), see Amoxil
Trinalin (pseudoephedrine and azatadine), 116–117
Triphasil (levonorgestrel and ethinyl estradiol), see Alesse-28
Triprolidine, pseudoephedrine and (Actifed), 134

Tryptophan, 205
Tums (calcium carbonate), 176
Tylenol, see also Acetaminophen
Tylenol Cold and Flu (acetaminophen, pseudoephedrine, and dextromethorphan), 177–178
Tylenol No. 3 (acetaminophen and codeine), 117
Tylenol PM (acetaminophen and diphenhydramine), 178–179
Tylenol Sinus (acetaminophen and pseudoephedrine), 179–180

U

Ulcerative colitis, treating, 20, 89–90
Ulcers, treating, 30, 96–97, 191, 200–201
Ultram (tramadol), 118
Umbilical cord, 7
Unisom (doxylamine), 180
Upper respiratory allergies, treating, 139
Upper respiratory tract inflammation, treating, 200–201
Upset stomach, treating, 158–159, 167, 191–192, 195, 199–201
Urinary problems, treating, 204, 206
Urinary tract infections, treating, 77–78, 100, 118–119, 199–200
Urine pregnancy tests, 1
Urine samples, morning, 2
Urised (methenamine, phenyl salicylate, methylene blue, benzoic acid, atropine, and hyoscyamine), 118–119
Uterus, 4
Uva Ursi, 206

V

Vaginal bacterial infections, treating, 37–38
Vaginal candidiasis, treating, 44–45
Vaginal yeast infections, treating, 156, 159
Vagistat-1 (tioconazole), 181
Valacyclovir (Valtrex), 119–120
Valerian, 206–207